Praise for Pavel Tsatsouline and for the First Edition of *Beyond Crunches*

"Thank you for the great job you did in your presentation (on abdominal training) at the **Arnold Fitness EXPO Seminar.** We received uniformly favorable comments concerning the quality of your instruction and the content of your message. As you know the fitness enthusiasts we attract to our seminars are very knowledgeable individuals. Hence, their supportive feedback concerning you and your presentation is of special significance."—*James J. Lorimer, Schwarzenegger/Lorimer Productions*

"The Pavelizer is the rage among the iron elite."—*Marty Gallagher, World Masters Powerlifting Champion, WashingtonPost.com*

"I am writing on behalf of the entire **Board of Directors of the Texas Tactical Police Officers Association** to express our sincere gratitude to you for helping with our Conference 2000. We trained 536 officers from 129 agencies.

Your portion of the instruction was a huge success. All of the student critiques were very complimentary. As a team leader with the **Houston Police Department SWAT team**, I am constantly looking for new ways to improve my physical performance. According to the student comments, you have truly introduced a new and revolutionary fitness program to our members.

In particular, our members commented on your common sense, practical exercises that utilize a minimum amount of equipment to achieve the very goals that other instructors require thousands of dollars of equipment to achieve. These techniques will help each officer reach new levels of fitness and ultimately improve their ability to protect the communities they serve.It is our mission to provide the very best training available, anywhere. Your efforts helped make that possible. "—*M.L. "Sandy" Wall, Training Advisor, TTPOZ*

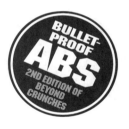

"I have seen many abdominal routines in the last 25 years and the *Beyond Crunches* program is the best yet."—*Steve Maxwell, M.Sc., Senior World Brazilian Jujitsu Champion*

"As a chiropractic physician, I see the deleterious effects of a weak torso on the lower back. Weak abs lead to years of back pain and dysfunction. As a world record holding powerlifter, I know the importance of strong abs on maximum power performance. *Beyond Crunches* is THE text and authority on ab/trunk stability."—*Dr. Fred Clary, National Powerlifting Champion and World Record Holder*

"I learned a lot from Pavel's books and video, and plan to use many of his ideas in my own workouts, especially the nontraditional ab exercises described in *Beyond Crunches*."—*Clarence Bass, Most Muscular Man, Mr. U.S.A, Past 40, author of Ripped 1, 2 & 3 and Lean for Life*

"Congratulations on your book *Beyond Crunches*. I found several of the insights and expressions to be very interesting and thought provoking (The Ab Pavelizer is just one). I will be implementing some of them into my own abdominal workout schedules."—*Dennis B. Weiss, author of Mass!, Raw Muscle & Anabolic Muscle Mass*

"Expect to find some of the most grueling stomach-busters that you have ever experienced—Tsatsouline advocates low-repetition intensity over high-repetition "burn" exercises, and introduces us to the Ab Pavelizer, a machine of his own invention that allows for perfect sit-ups. *Beyond Crunches* has many new and challenging drills, making this a great manual for anyone who needs some variety in their workout routine. Included is the Flag, Bruce Lee's favorite abdominal exercise."—*Brendan J. LaSalle, Amazon.com*

"As someone who has been crippled twice by injuries to my spine and had to rebuild my body from scratch twice, I have two things to say: 1) serious abdominal conditioning is *mandatory* for anyone with back pain and anyone who intends to push their body in sport or martial arts and 2) Pavel's book is, by far, the best book I've seen on this vitally important and neglected subject." —*Ken McCarthy, New York*

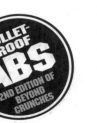

"This book took me from having a back that everyone told me was too weak to ever do heavy lifting and that was in almost constant pain to no back pain and new PR's in the deadlift and Squat. Pavel's ab exercises are the stuff champions are made of. Clear, concise directions and radical new ideas make this book well worth the money spent. And it's for every trainee with a desire to succeed. I've heard that you must already be very advanced to begin the exercises in this book, but I recently began training my 50 year old father-in-law using these techniques and after about a month he was doing Janda situps with the best of them. Not to mention he no longer complains of back pain and has better posture. Get this book and throw out all of your others on abs!"
—*Chris Dudzik, Hollister, CA.*

"Pavel delivers once again! This book details the mechanics of abdominal and oblique development in an easy to understand, user-friendly format. Learn to either build up your midsection, tone it up, get a prominent six-pack, and/or increase your punching and throwing power by learning to integrate your powerful midsection! There is one particular exercise that I found to be super productive in adding to punching power, and this is the only book that has it... It is extremely simple and easy to understand. Pavel explains how to protect your spine and perform the "perfect" situp. All in all a great book by a great author, definitely a must-have for any fighter and lifter. My punching power and deadlifting strength went up very quickly on this program and I am very pleased."— *Sean Williams, Long Beach, NY*

"I've bought the TV advertised training devices and a bundle of ab books—tried them all. But, doing the routines Pavel Tsatsouline presents in this book is the way I have achieved solid abs! Pavel offers a great deal of knowledge in an easy to digest manner. His writing, while colloquial, is founded in research and deep understanding of physiology and kinesthetics. I highly recommend this book."— *Linda Crawford, Minnesota State Masters Powerlifting Champion and Record Holder, Minneapolis, MN*

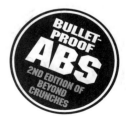

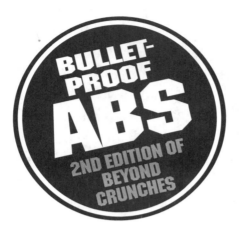

Published in the United States by:
Dragon Door Publications, Inc

P.O. Box 4381, St. Paul, MN 55104
Tel: (651) 487-2180 • Fax: (651) 487-3954
Credit card orders: 1-800-899-5111
Email: dragondoor@aol.com • Website: www.dragondoor.com

ISBN: 0-938045-25-3

Book design, Illustrations and cover by Derek Brigham
Website http//www.dbrigham.com
Tel/Fax: (612) 827-3431 • Email: dbrigham@visi.com
Digital photography by Andrea Du Cane and
Robert Pearl Photography • Tel: (612) 617-7724

Manufactured in the United States
Third Edition: April 2002

DISCLAIMER
The author and publisher of this material are not responsible in any manner whatsoever for any injury that may occur through following the instructions contained in this material. The activities, physical and otherwise, described herein for informational purposes only, may be too strenuous or dangerous for some people and the reader(s) should consult a physician before engaging in them.

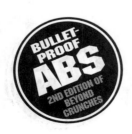

Dedication

To my parents, Ella and Vladimir,
as an apology for not becoming
a rocket scientist.

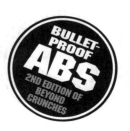

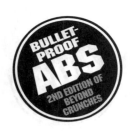

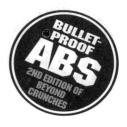

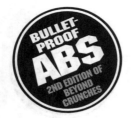

Part I
How to Truly Isolate Your Abs—for Faster, More Effective Results

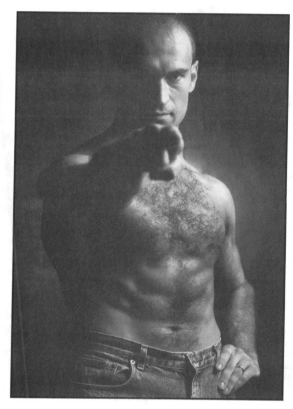

Comrade! I have forged bullet-proof abs for the Special Forces of the Evil Russian Empire. You are next! If you don't know how—I'll teach you. If you don't want to—I'll make you.

I am Pavel. I forged bullet-proof abs for the crack troops of the Evil Soviet Empire. You are next! If you don't know how—I'll teach you. If you don't want to—I'll make you.

While crunches rival baseball as the national pastime and infomercial ab gizmos are selling like hot dogs, an average American gut still looks more like an air bag than a six-pack. I'll fix it.

It is universally accepted that the perfect ab exercise:

1) maximizes isolation of the abdominal muscles;

2) reduces lower back stress by minimizing the involvement of the hip flexors (the psoas group);

3) fool-proofs itself by the nature of its performance.

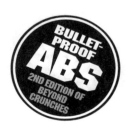

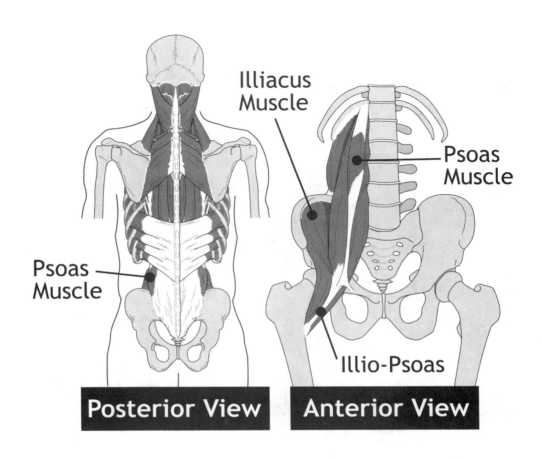

Illiacus Muscle

Psoas Muscle

Psoas Muscle

Illio-Psoas

Posterior View

Anterior View

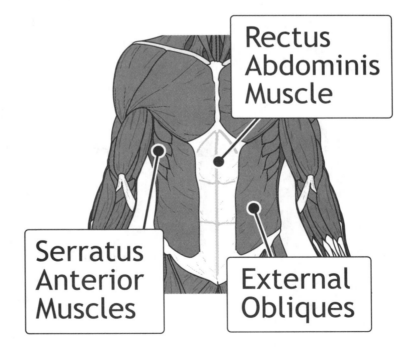

Rectus Abdominis Muscle

Serratus Anterior Muscles

External Obliques

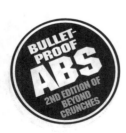

Before accepting the solution, you must understand the problem.

The abdominals *(rectus abdominis)* connect your pubic bone to your breast bone. When this muscle contracts, it pulls your pelvis and rib cage together, rounding your back in the process, as in a crunch. This is called 'forward spinal flexion'. (Fig. 1)

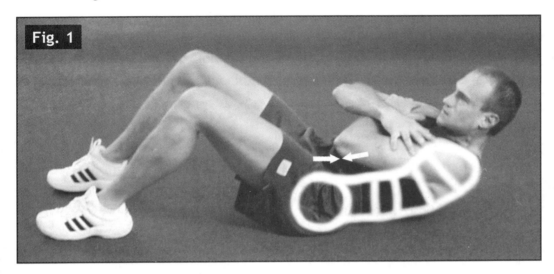

Fig. 1

Psoas major originates on the vertebrae of the lower back, and inserts into the top of the thigh bone. When this muscle contracts, it pulls the body into a jackknife position. When you do a situp, you literally pull yourself up by your lumbar spine, or lower back (Fig. 2)—which can lead to back problems or aggravate the existing ones.

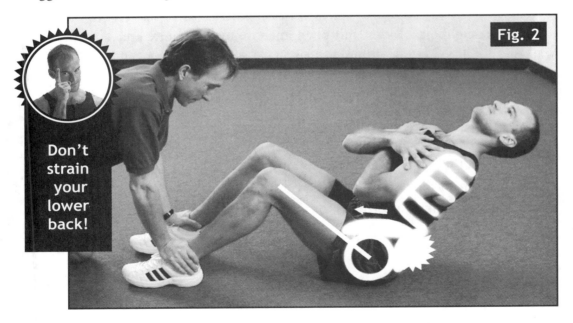

Fig. 2

Don't strain your lower back!

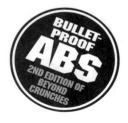

A common so called 'solution' is to avoid hip flexion, or situps, and do only spinal flexion, or crunches. A number of gizmos were designed to capitalize on the public obsession with crunches. All of them were supposed to make crunches stricter. The *Ab Isolator* immobilized the hip joint; the *AbFlex* increased the recruitment of the abdominals during the crunch by providing direct pressure on the muscles; the *AbRoller* tracked the crunch mechanically.

There are two problems with these products. First, they are gimmicks. According to John Jakicic, Ph.D., an exercise physiologist and assistant professor at the University of Pittsburgh School of Medicine, these devices "offer no physiological advantage over doing crunches with good form."

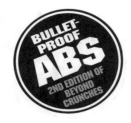

The second problem is the crunch itself. Contrary to the popular opinion, the crunch does NOT isolate the abs. Ditto for any crunch based device. Because the crunch does not involve hip flexion, it supposedly does not involve the psoas group and stress the lower back. Wrong.

Well known physical therapists Kendall, Kendall, and Wadsworth determined that it is impossible to completely eliminate the hip flexor recruitment during a crunch. One of the fundamental laws of physiology, the *Law of Irradiation*, dictates that the contraction of a muscle, the abdominals in this case, will set off a contraction of the adjacent muscles, or the hip flexors. Like a stone dropped in the water sends ripples across the surface, tension spreads—irradiates—from the muscle directly responsible for the job at hand towards its neighbors. To test this phenomenon, make a white knuckle fist. Your biceps will tense up, although there is no movement in the elbow joint!

According to John Scaringe, D.C., the president of the American Chiropractic Board of Sports Physicians, a person with weak abdominals relies on his or her stronger hip flexors even during crunches. The trainee cannot get his torso off the floor by rounding his back with his abs, so he yanks on his spine with his hip flexors to gain momentum! (Fig. 3) It does not take an Einstein to figure out that such training is worthless for the abs and dangerous to the spine.

Fig. 3

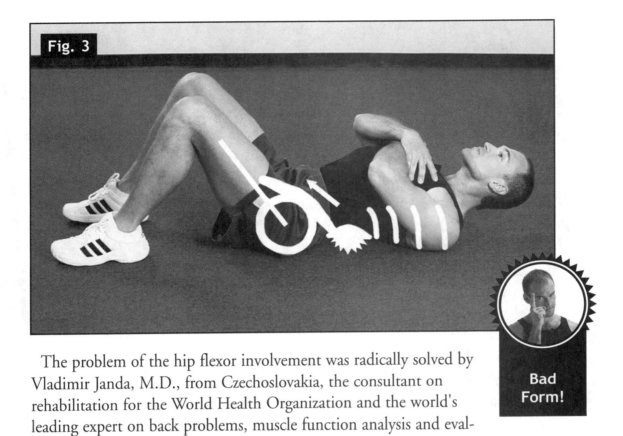

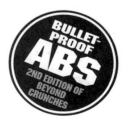

Bad Form!

The problem of the hip flexor involvement was radically solved by Vladimir Janda, M.D., from Czechoslovakia, the consultant on rehabilitation for the World Health Organization and the world's leading expert on back problems, muscle function analysis and evaluation.

Professor Janda relaxed the psoas group using another neurological phenomenon: the *Law of Reciprocal Inhibition.* When a muscle contracts, its antagonist, or the opposite number, relaxes. It is about efficiency. The alternative would be similar to stepping on the gas and the brake simultaneously.

Dr. Janda had his patient assume the standard bent knee situp/crunch position and placed his hands under the latter's calves. The patient attempted to sit up while steadily pushing against the doctor's hands. This activated the knee flexor and hip extensor muscles (the hamstrings and glutes). Reciprocal inhibition took place and the hip flexors relaxed. **The result: back stress was eliminated and the abdominals were isolated!** (Fig. 4)

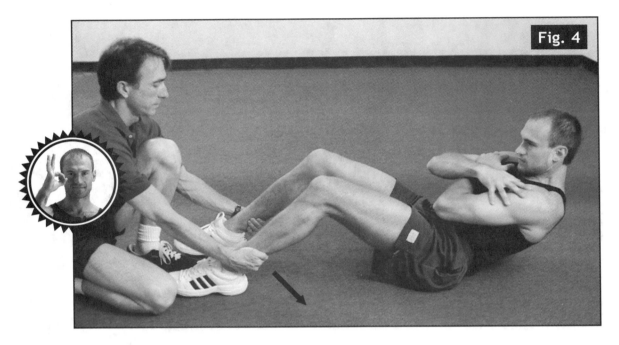

Fig. 4

Until recently the Janda situp could not be performed without a training partner. Although the professor recommended pressing into the wall with the toes and simultaneously down into floor (Fig. 5), *it does not work*. It is very tempting to leg press the wall instead of pulling down. This is exactly what a trainee will do when he gets tired. Then the contraction of the quads engages the hip flexors next door, thanks to the good ol' Law of Irradiation.

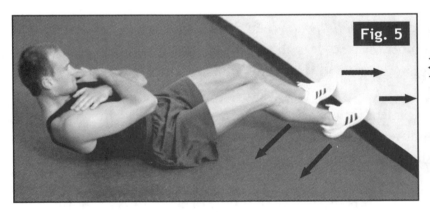

Fig. 5

Not reliable!

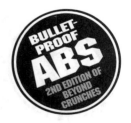

Pushing through the floor with one's heels or feet, as in 'the crunch with active prepositioning', proposed by chiropractors Jerry Hyman and Craig Liebenson, is also ineffective because of poor leverage. The muscular tension—and training effect—is minimal (Fig. 6A, 6B). Ditto for crunches with your paws up on a bench.

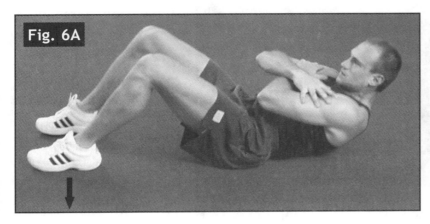

Fig. 6A

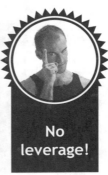

No leverage!

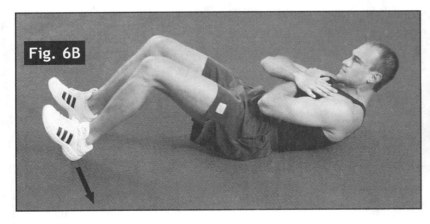

Fig. 6B

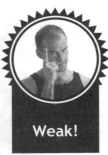

Weak!

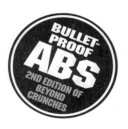

The Ab Pavelizer™

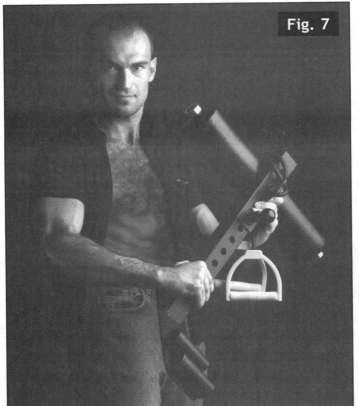

Fig. 7

Enter the Ab Pavelizer™. This new product allows the performance of the Janda situp without a training partner (Fig. 7). In fact, it is more comfortable because the trainee regulates the pressure, rather than the training partner.

This portable new device fits under a door and provides comfortable padded rollers to push against with the back of your legs while doing Janda situps. It comes with is a bungee cord

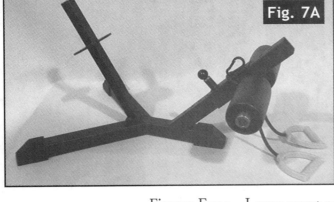

Fig. 7A

with handles to assist the individuals who are too weak to perform the exercise—which means most people!

When I challenged the audience at a recent Arnold's Seminar to do five strict Janda situps, a husky bodybuilder who came onstage barely managed two reps! I repeated the challenge when I returned to my booth at Arnold Schwarzenegger Fitness Expo. I even went as far as promising to print the names of the tough cookies who managed a fiver on the Ab Pavelizer™ in my column in a bodybuilding magazine. Many world class bodybuilders, powerlifters, and martial artists tried—and only a handful earned the fame!

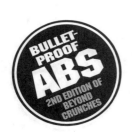

According to Joseph Horrigan, D.C., of the Soft Tissue Center in Los Angeles, two or three Janda situps are considered to be 'good'. When you do a set of Janda situps to the limit, the high level of difficulty and the extreme isolation of the abs are obvious.

After performing a Janda, then immediately hook your feet under a couch and do a standard situp. You will find that you can do many—easily. Doing Ab Pavelizer™ situps back to back with crunches—with or without any flaky crunch gizmo—is also a revelation. The tension you feel in the abs is clearly superior with the new machine. The crunch belongs on the junk pile of history next to communism! The movement is just too subtle to generate high tension in the target muscles.

If you do not have an Ab Pavelizer™ yet, call (800) 899-5111 to get it, and let's start rocking!

How do I use my Ab Pavelizer™?

Open a door and slide the device underneath. You may want to place a towel between the door and your Ab Pavelizer™ to protect the former from being damaged by the industrial steel machine. No cheap imported plastic here, Comrade! There is enough metal in an Ab Pavelizer™ to forge an *RPK*, or a Kalashnikov machine gun!

Shut the door—and make sure that no one tries to open it! Lie on the floor, the way you used to for crunches, and place your calves atop the roller pads. Do not wear pants made of slippery fabric like nylon or your calves will slide off the roller pads (Fig. 8). You may also end up dragging your butt toward the machine.

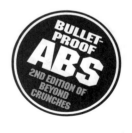

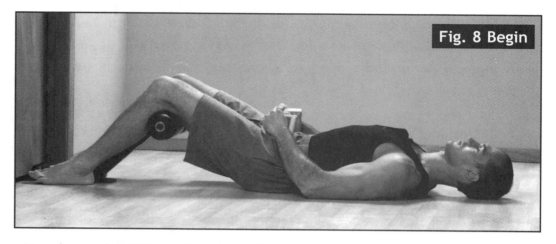

Fig. 8 Begin

Your knees should be at the ninety-degree angle—square at the corner —and the pads should hit you about half way between your ankles and your knees. Adjust them accordingly.

Ab Pavelizer™ situps are difficult and your best bet is to start by doing 'negatives', or only the lowering half of the drill. Sit upright with your knees at a ninety-degree angle, your calves touching the pads, and your feet flat on the floor (Fig. 9).

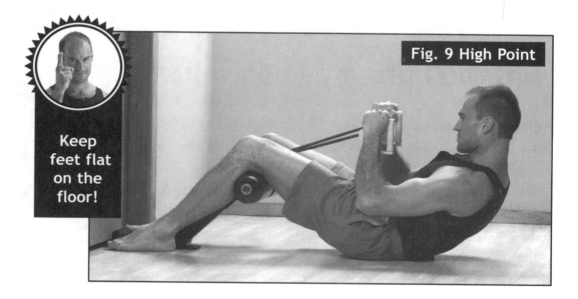

Fig. 9 High Point

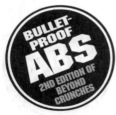

Keep feet flat on the floor!

Keep your arms nearly straight and your hands on the floor by your sides. Take a normal breath, squeeze your butt as hard as you can, and slowly lower yourself to the ground **WHILE MAINTAINING THE TENSION IN THE GLUTES**, keeping your feet down and exerting pressure against the roller pads—as if you are pawing the ground. Initially you may have trouble keeping your feet down. It will pass.

Descend slowly, especially during the last couple of inches above the ground. You will only be able to do so if your keep your glutes tight! Take three to four seconds to get all the way down. Keep your chin tucked in until your shoulders touch the floor. Stay tight until your head reaches the floor.

In the beginning it is a good idea to hold on to the bungee cord for extra assistance; Ab Pavelizer™ situps are a lot more challenging than they look! We have installed a bungee cord rather than some solid object to hold on to because a rubber band gives you immediate feedback on the amount of help you are getting. The more assistance you need, the closer to the device you should grab the cords. Hold your breath when you are in motion—unless your doctor told you otherwise (Fig. 10). In this and other drills where holding the breath is recommended, it is OK to take a mini breath of air here and there as long as it is barely noticeable and the abs stay tight.

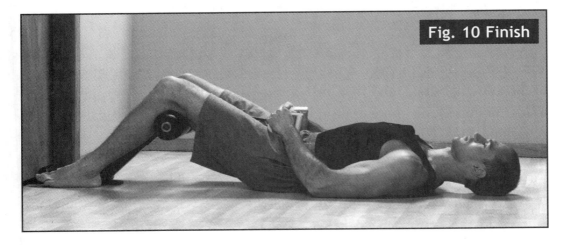

Fig. 10 Finish

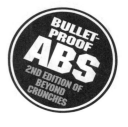

Once you have reached the bottom, rest your head on the floor and totally relax for a few seconds. Get up in any comfortable manner that is not hard on your body, for example rolling off to the side or helping with your arms. Do three to five sets of three to five reps with three to five minutes of rest in between. 3-5, it's easy to remember!

You can Pavelize your abs daily, but you will also get good results from every other day training. Once you can easily do 5x5 (five sets of five reps), bend your elbows and hold your fists by your face like a boxer. The next stage is holding your arms straight over your head. Once this stage is mastered, it is time to do the full drill, down and up!

After the first negative, relax, then take a normal breath, squeeze your glutes, and SLOWLY get up while keeping your glutes flexed and your feet flat. Once you have reached the upright position, exhale and relax. Feel free to rest for a couple of seconds, then inhale and perform the negative as described earlier.

It should take you three to four seconds to get up. It is not just a safety measure. You cannot have a high level of muscular tension if you move fast; therefore you will not gain much strength or muscle tone. It is much better to move slowly through the full range of the exercise with the humbling assistance of the bungee cord than to mindlessly knock off quick reps!

As before, start with the easiest version of the Ab Pavelizer™ situp, with your arms by your sides, and even holding on to the bungee cord, eventually work up to the 'boxer' position, and then the arms overhead position. One option is to lower yourself in a more challenging position than the one you used for getting up.

If even the most challenging position becomes easy, hold a light barbell plate or something like a soup can in your straight arms. Even if you are a stud, don't scoff at the soup can; it may take you a long time to work up to it!

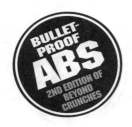

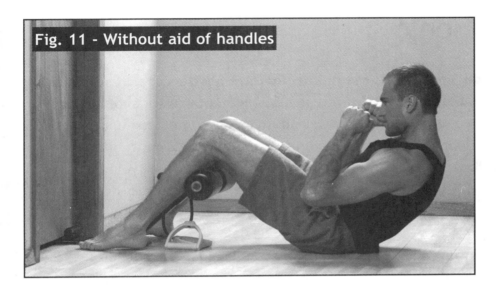

Fig. 11 - Without aid of handles

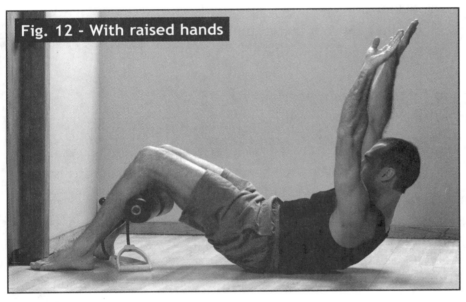

Fig. 12 - With raised hands

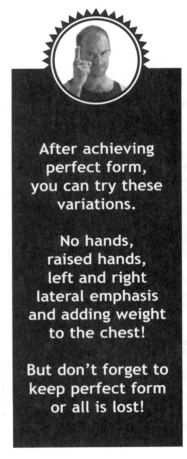

After achieving perfect form, you can try these variations.

No hands, raised hands, left and right lateral emphasis and adding weight to the chest!

But don't forget to keep perfect form or all is lost!

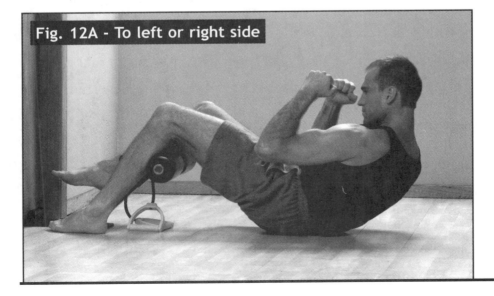

Fig. 12A - To left or right side

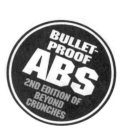

Questions:

When I do 'negatives', I can do the top three quarters of the movement very slowly, then I just 'fall through' near the floor. What should I do?

Pace yourself so it takes you 3-4 seconds to evenly go from the upright position to the floor, rather than taking four seconds for the top part of the drill only to collapse to the bottom in a fraction of a second. Keep your glutes locked tight. Consider getting some assistance from the bungee cords for the last hard inches.

On the way down on the last rep of every set you may also hold on to the bungee cord and pause for a 1-5 seconds at your weak angle. You will quickly strengthen your sticking point with this powerful Russian technique. If you choose to use it, do not hold your breath during the pause! Make the breath shallow and constrained to maintain steady intra-abdominal pressure.

Do I have to try to curl and uncurl my back?

As long as you move slowly, without jerks, Ab Pavelizer™ situps will take care of the proper lower back alignment. Your back will curl without you having to worry about it.

My lower back muscles feel tight when I do Ab Pavelizer™ situps. Any suggestions?

Prof. Janda recommends stretching your lower back if you have this problem. I recommend a souped up toe touch. Stand with your back close to wall. Do not touch the wall, it is there to spot you if you lose balance.

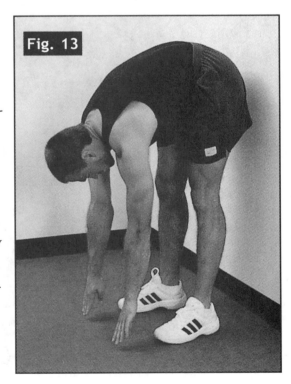

Fig. 13

Keeping your knees locked or nearly locked, slowly bend over as far as you can. (Fig.13) Next, inhale and tighten up the muscles on the rear side of your body: your back, glutes, and hamstrings.

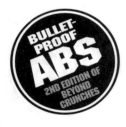

Imagine your body is a tightly clenched fist. Hold the tension— and your breath—for a second, then suddenly relax and let the air out with tension. You will drop an inch or two increasing your stretch.

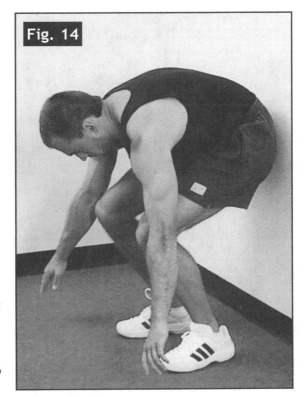

Fig. 14

I like the graphic description of this tension/release sequence by Dr. Judd Biasiotto:

"You must relax instantly... picture yourself exerting all your strength in an effort to push a large boulder off a sheer cliff. When suddenly the boulder goes over the edge, there is no active resistance to your pushing and all you straining instantly ceases. It is that feeling, that nothingness after the boulder drops, that you are striving to obtain when you "turn off your source of power".

Sigh with relief, and repeat. When you can no longer increase the stretch, bend your knees, and stand up. (Fig. 14) Bending your knees on the way up is essential. It relieves the distress on your back making the once criticized toe touch a safer back stretch.

If you want to know more about state of the art Russian stretching methods, *Power Stretching* is the book for you. **Call (800) 899-5111** and regain the buoyant flexibility of your youth.

I have a serious back condition. Can I do Ab Pavelizer™ situps?
Only with your doctor's approval. Chances are that you will get it. Ab Pavelizer™ situps are surprisingly easy on the lower back. Usually Comrades with bad backs report that their backs feel AWESOME from Ab Pavelizer™ situps—even if they hurt from any other ab drill, including crunches.

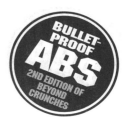

My neck usually bothers me when I train my abs. Will this be a problem with Ab Pavelizer™ situps?

Not likely. We only do three to five reps per set, that is not long enough to exhaust your neck muscles. Besides, you are supposed to take a brief rest every time you lie down and sit up. Also, do not place your hands behind your neck.

Do I have to sit all the way up? I heard that you only work your abs as you come off the floor.

Even though the original Janda situp takes you only half the way up, I instruct my victims to sit all the way up. You will get an extra break on the top that will translate into greater concentration on tension and better gains in muscle tone.

Does the Ab Pavelizer™ strengthen and tone all the muscles of my mid-section?

You bet, Comrade! Prof. Janda did EMG tests of his supersitup and it showed increased electrical activity in both the abs and the obliques. For extra emphasis on your obliques, or the 'love handle' muscles, I recommend you descend with most of your weight on one foot (you don't need to twist). Alternate your sides every rep, for example left-right-left-right for a four rep set or left-right-left-right-straight for five repetitions. Do not use this technique until you have mastered the basic Ab Pavelizer™ situp(Fig.12A).

Will the Ab Pavelizer™ make me a better athlete, or are my newly shredded abs just for looks?

I have never compromised function for form in my training programs. Pavelized abs are as strong as they look.

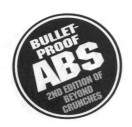

What can I expect?

OK, so you go toe to toe with the Ab Pavelizer™. You blitz your abs into screaming submission. You temper your laughable belly into a bunched pack of knuckle-breaking nasties. You startle yourself when you catch your abs in the mirror. You'd cause the Terminator to go into meltdown.

Fine. But can you handle the rest of it? From people?—the fear? The respect? The envy? The blatant desire? The worship? Get a grip now—we are talking serious emotional situations.

Can you handle just being for your abs? Can you handle the constant staring? The wanting? The popeyed disbelief? The whispering behind your back? Rubberneckers getting into fender benders at the sight of you? If you are going to have Pavelized abs you better be able to handle the attention. It gives a whole new meaning to 'gut-check time'. If you can't hack it, then get help— and order your Ab Pavelizer™ when you are ready.

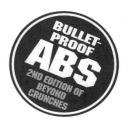

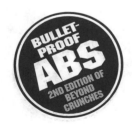

Part II
Integration: How to Turn Your Abs into Team Players—and Skyrocket Your Athletic Potential

A few years ago James Garrick, M.D., tested the abdominal strength of the U.S. junior national gymnastics team. None of these athletes, whose muscle definition, according to Dr. Garrick, "strained belief", and a number of whom went on to represent the United States in the upcoming summer Olympics, could do five crunches!

Dr. Garrick, who happened to be the medical advisor to the NFL, the U.S. Figure Skating Team, and the San Francisco Ballet, correctly identified the problem: "It wasn't that they didn't have muscles... it was just that these muscles weren't functioning as back stabilizers. They were doing other things. When they were called into play... they weren't equal to the job."

Most people do not realize that having muscle is not the same thing as being strong. If that was the case, weightlifting competition would end at the weigh-in and bodybuilders would collect all the trophies.

Explains Professor Vladimir Zatsiorsky, a former strength and conditioning consultant to Soviet Olympic teams:

"Maximal force exertion is a skilled action where many muscles must be appropriately activated. This coordinated activation of many muscle groups is called intermuscular coordination."

In plain English, take a bunch of good football players who have never played as a team, throw them out on the field, and watch them getting whipped!

Bullet-Proof Abs is a comprehensive two step program. The first step was isolation, or <u>training the muscles</u>. Janda situps have isolated your abs from the hip flexors to strengthen and tone them in the quickest, most efficient manner.

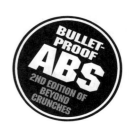

Next step is integration, or <u>training the movement</u>. The following drills will not only tone up your soft underbellies, but will teach them how to work as a team with other muscles and protect your spine.

The primary function of the abs is not to pull your ribcage and your pelvis together—unless you are a crunch junkie or you chop firewood for a living—but to provide a stable platform for other muscles to pull from.   For instance, tensed abdominals balance the pull of the psoas on the spine—thus maintaining its normal curve.

When a person runs, lifts or kicks without the requisite strength ratio between spine flexor and hip flexor, the hip flexors will arch the lower back—and possibly injure it. (Fig. 15)

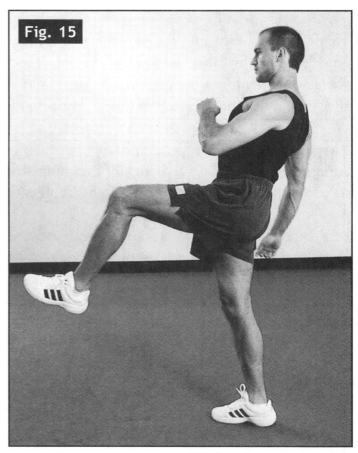

Fig. 15

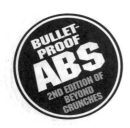

A pole is a helpful analogy. Supported with guy wires (psoas) on one side, it will bend, break, or fall. (Fig. 16) Add another set of cables (abs) on the other side, and the post will be more stable than ever. (Fig. 17)

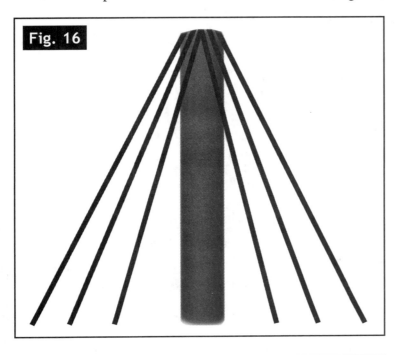

Fig. 16

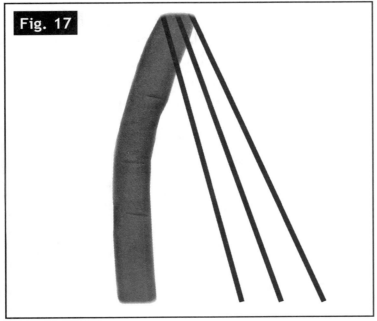

Fig. 17

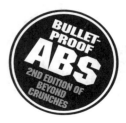

So after you have developed your abdominal muscles with Ab Pavelizert™ situps, train your hip flexors and your abs to work as a team. Here is the drill.

The Russian Ballet Leg Thrust

Gymnasts and dancers overdevelop their hip flexors with all the leg raises they do. Eventually, in spite of all their splits and stretches, these muscles shorten (If you are curious why it happens, why relaxed stretching cannot help it, and what can be done about it—check out *Power Stretching*, the book.) They pull on the spine, inducing unhealthy hyperlordosis, or an exaggerated arch of the lower back.

Russian ballet dancers and gymnasts favor the drill I am about to describe because it trains the abs to stabilize their spines against their powerful hip flexors. This exercise also overloads the interspinales, deep muscles of the back, important for spinal health. In the process you will develop corrugated abs you will be proud of.

Start working one leg at a time. Lie on your back with one leg pointed straight at the ceiling—or its neighborhood, depending on your flexibility—and the other parked a la fossilized crunch. (Fig. 18) Flatten your lower back against the floor and keep it there for the duration of the set.

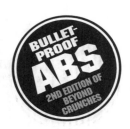

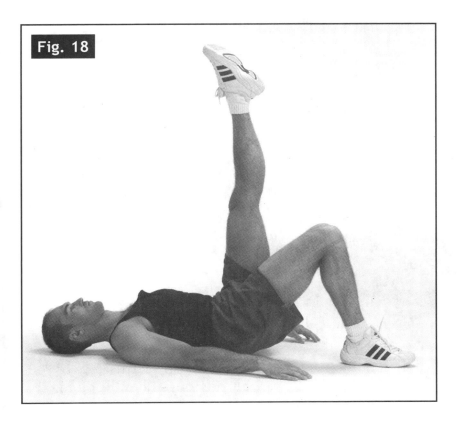

Fig. 18

Inhale, squeeze your butt, and slowly lower your leg. Keep your toes pointed, and go down as low as you can while keeping your lumbar spine flat. Stop short of creating any discomfort in the small of your back. (Fig. 19) It is easy to let your back go concave without you realizing it. Initially, when you are learning the Russian Ballet Leg Thrust, have somebody try to slide a pen under your back. They should not be able to.

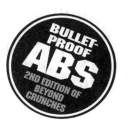

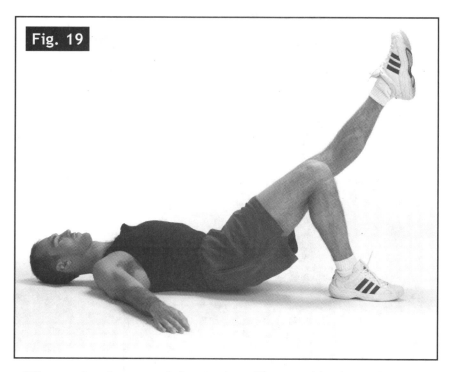

Fig. 19

The tension in your abdominals will invariably drop if you breathe during this exercise, giving your hip flexors an opportunity to overpower your abs and possibly causing a back injury. That means that if your doctor disapproves breath holding during exercise–you have been excused from this drill, Comrade.

If you are forced to reverse the movement before you have reached the ground, keep holding your breath until you get back up then release it and relax for a second before the next repetition. If you have successfully lowered your paw to the floor (Fig. 20), park it and relax for a second before inhaling and heading back up. Work one side for the required number of reps—three to five—then take care of the other.

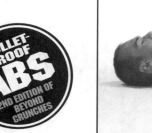

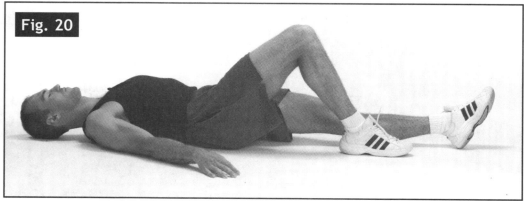

Fig. 20

As you improve, gradually straighten out your planted leg until it is flat on the floor (Fig. 21 & 22). At this point you may add an ankle weight or switch to the two-legged version.

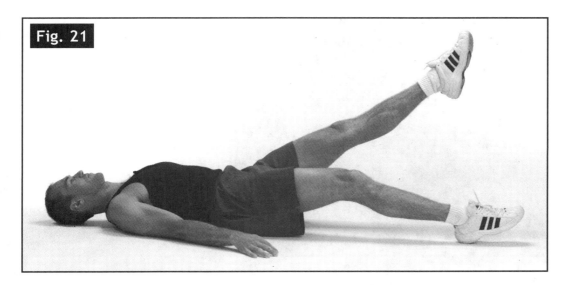

Fig. 21

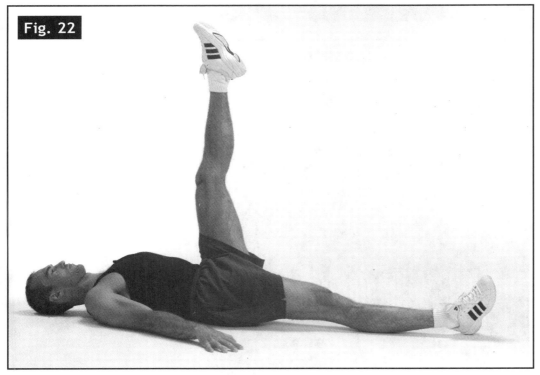

Fig. 22

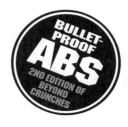

Lie down on your back and bring your knees towards your chest (Fig. 23), then follow the instructions for the one legged version of this evil drill.

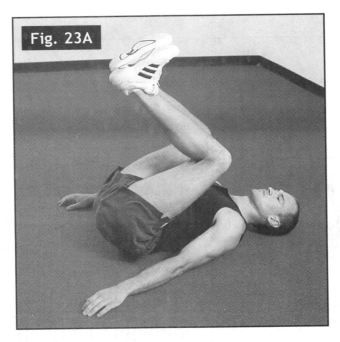

Fig. 23A

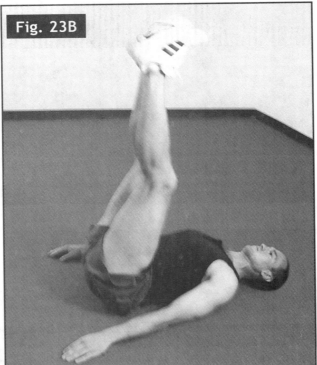

Fig. 23B

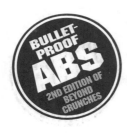

If you are having trouble with this exercise, you could try an easier version, with your spine flexed forward, as in a crunch, and your head up. (Fig. 24)

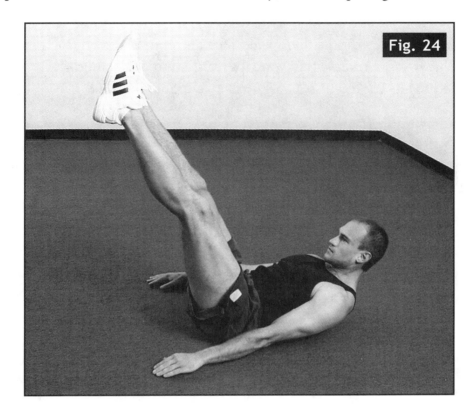

Fig. 24

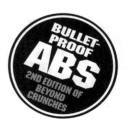

Situps—the Right Way

Here is a test to see if you are ready for situps. You must be able to flatten your back against the floor while keeping your legs straight on the floor. (Fig. 25) If you cannot, either your abs are still too weak, and/or your hip flexors are too tight. Lacking the intermuscular coordination could also be a problem.

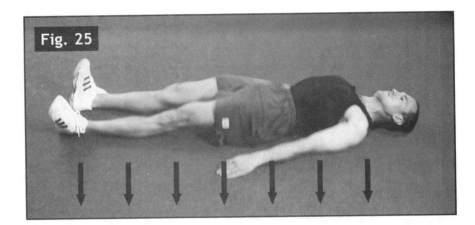

Fig. 25

Keep Pavelizing your budding six-pack with Janda situps, practice pressing your back into the floor from a crunch position, (Fig. 26), and stretch your hip flexors. I do not need to remind you which book has the flexibility know-how, or, as one confused Russian engineer would say, 'go-home'. He also called his green card 'green peace', in case you care.

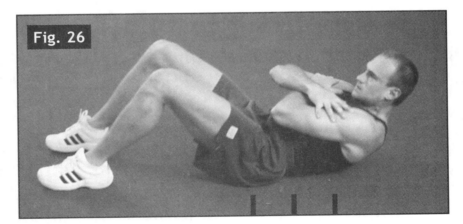

Fig. 26

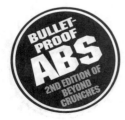

Conventional situps (Fig. 27) have to be modified to be made safer and more effective. First, the hip flexors should be worked through a longer range of motion to avoid adaptive shortening and consequent back and posture problems. Your hips and torso should be in a straight line at the starting point of a situp as in straight-legged situps. (Fig. 28) However, if your lower back and hamstring flexibility is poor, you will not be able to perform straight-legged situps properly. Practice the stretch described in conjunction with the Ab Pavelizer™ and do your situps with your knees bent to relax your hamstrings.

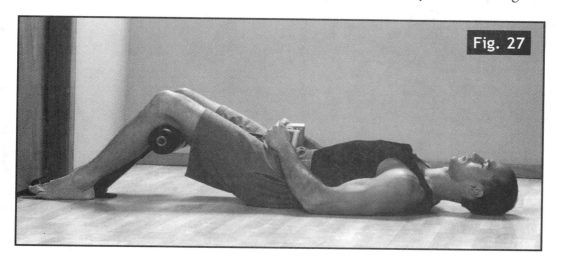

Fig. 27

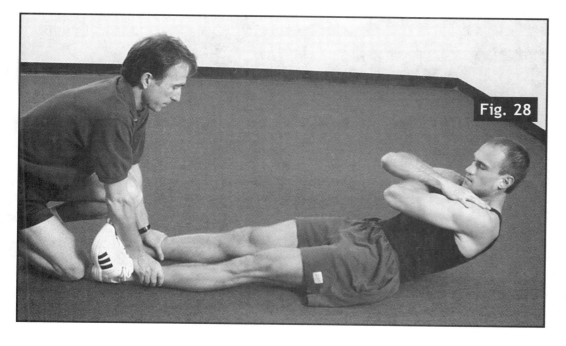

Fig. 28

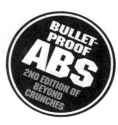

Exercise on a situp board (Fig. 29), or you can use a table and anchor your feet around its legs. Having a training partner hold your feet down is also fine. If you use a decline bench (Fig. 30A), you will be able to overload your abs even better.

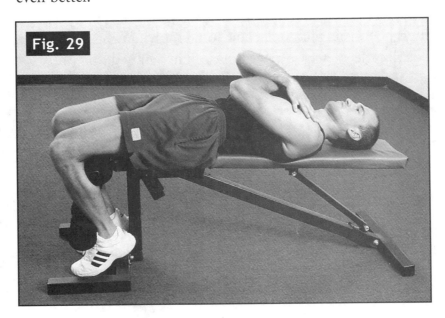

Fig. 29

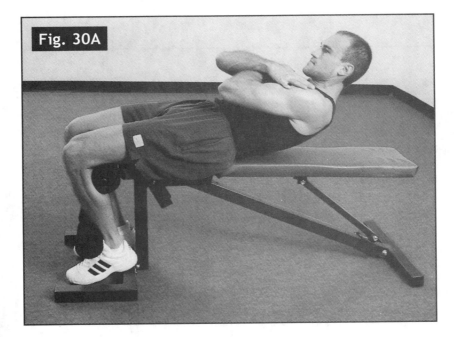

Fig. 30A

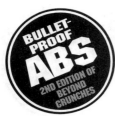

Fold your hands on your chest, with an extra weight if possible, inhale, and flatten your back against the bench as you have in the situp test. Maintaining this back alignment, sit up smoothly (Fig. 30B) all the way to the top. Semi-relax, make sure your lumbar spine is flat or rounded—it is very important!—and lower yourself all the way down. Exhale, relax for a moment, repeat.

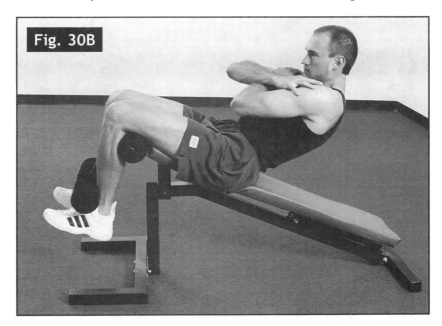

Fig. 30B

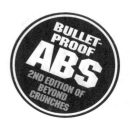

When you work up to a heavy weight, barbell plates or dumbbells will be too awkward to use. Holding a barbell near your collar bones will work better. (Fig. 30C)

Prof. Anatoly Laputin of the Kiev Physical Culture Institute in the Ukraine recommended a simple yet highly effective variation of the straight-legged situp. I was told that Pilates practitioners perform a very similar exercise.

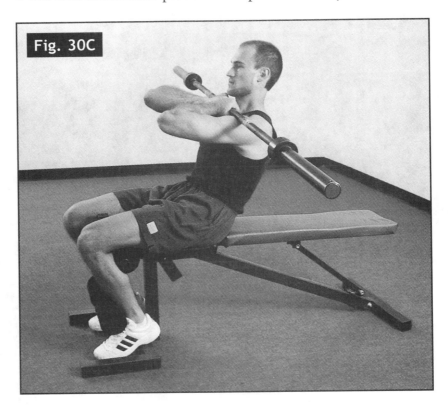

Fig. 30C

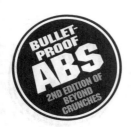

Lie on your back with your arms along your body. (Fig. 31) Inhale, flatten your back by squeezing your butt, and slowly roll up your spine starting with your neck and working down to your thoracic, and finally lumbar spine. (Fig. 32) You may visualize wrapping your head in your torso in the beginning of the movement. Reach out to your toes with your pointed fingers as you are curling up. Go as far as possible (Fig. 33) working against the increasing resistance of the hamstrings, spinal erectors, and the viscera. In addition to strengthening the abs, this drill improves your flexibility and provides a healthy massage of your inner organs.

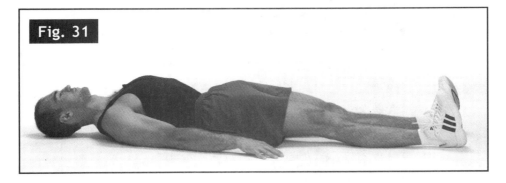

Fig. 31

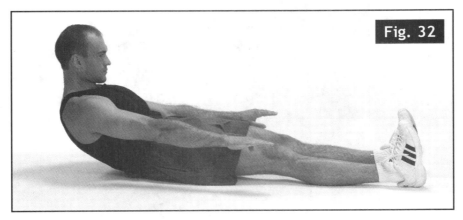

Fig. 32

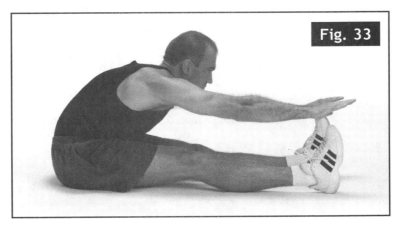

Fig. 33

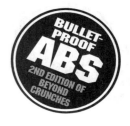

Relax when you reach your flexibility limit. Inhale, tense your glutes, and reverse the movement. You may use bungee cords for extra resistance but not weights. (Fig. 34-36) By the way, you may employ bungee cords in the same fashion with other situp variations.

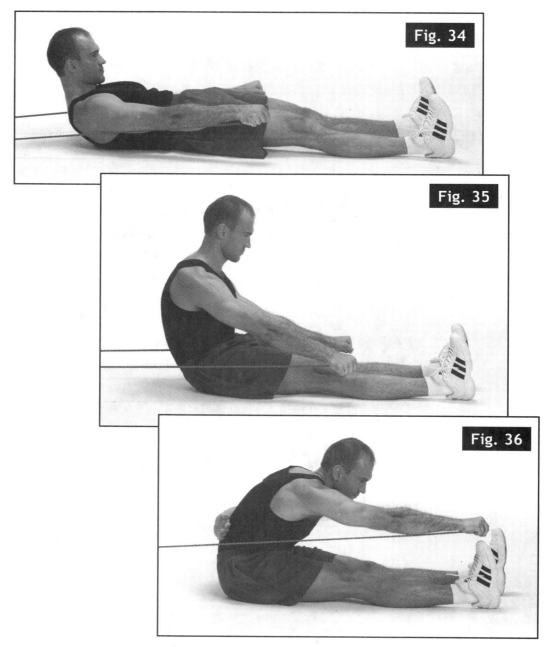

Fig. 34

Fig. 35

Fig. 36

"It is not a difficult exercise," comments A. N. Laputin, D. Sc., "But a highly effective one; its frequent repetition assures very rapid development of the abdominal muscles."

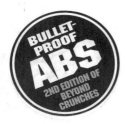

Scissor Situps

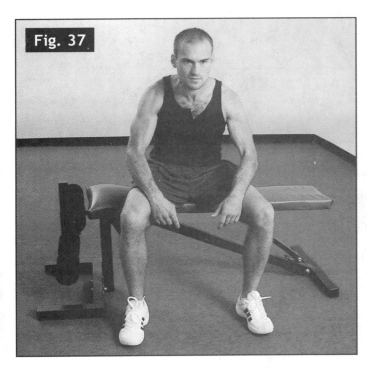

Fig. 37

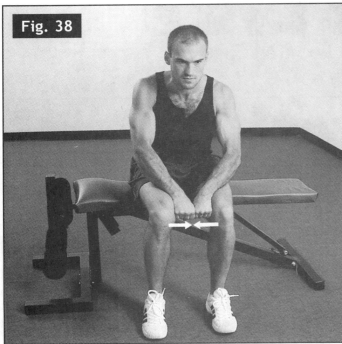

Fig. 38

Try an experiment. Sit in a chair with your hands on your knees and flex your abs as hard as possible. (Fig. 37)

Now put your fists inside your knees and do the same while squeezing your fists hard with your knees. (Fig. 38) You will see that your abs contract much stronger when you are trying to close your legs. Martial artists have been taking advantage of this phenomenon for centuries with strong stances like Okinawan karate's *sanchin-dachi*. This neat phenomenon, later rediscovered by the East Germans, enables us to design a state of the art situp.

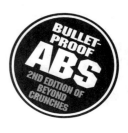

Lie down on an exercise bench or a narrow table with your knees bent to relieve your back. (Fig. 39) As with the conventional situps, if your strength and flexibility are up to snuff, you can do the drill straight-legged on the floor. (Fig. 40)

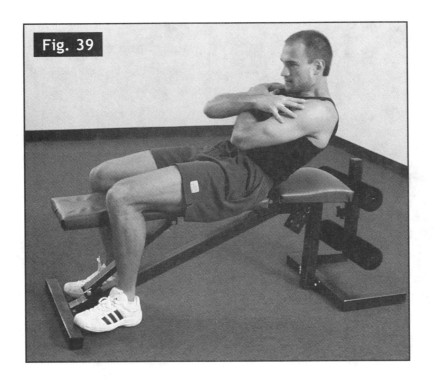

Fig. 39

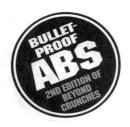

Follow every direction given for the regular situps, plus pinch the bench—or whatever you are using—with your knees, or ankles. Keep the muscles surrounding your knees tight. Make sure not to let your knees bow in or twist if you are doing the straight-legged version (Fig. 41)! If you cannot help it or have bad knees, stick to the bent-legged scissor situp, which should not torque your knees.

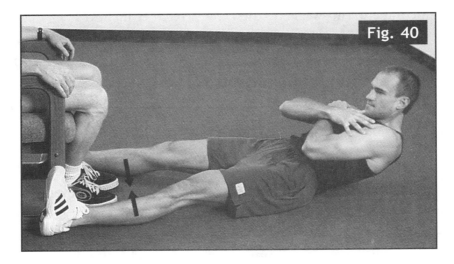

Fig. 40

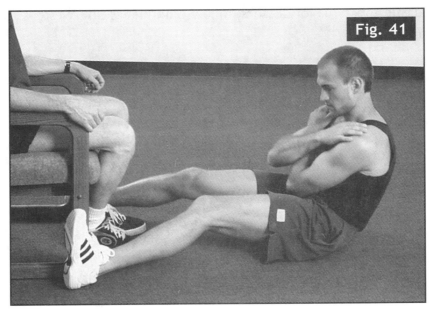

Fig. 41

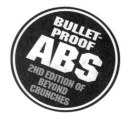

Swiss Ball Crunches

Recall that crunches are worthless because the movement is too subtle to generate sufficient tension in the abs. It is a different ball game if you double the range of motion of the crunch by placing some sort of a pad under your lower back and glutes. Dr. Fred Hatfield, the first man to squat over 1,000 pounds in competition, swears by these 'pre-stretch crunches'.

Stretching the abs amplified the intensity of their contraction and made the movement harder to confuse with head bobbing and spine yanking. Another plus is strengthening the abdominals in a stretched position—where they are often called to perform in sports.

Last but not least, performing at least some of your abdominal strength training in the stretched position helps your posture: you prevent the abs from shortening and giving you a hump. Now it should not surprise you that Russians, Olympic champions, health superstar Academician Amosov, and my aunt Inna, have been doggedly performing extreme stretch situps over a stool or some gymnastic apparatus for decades, totally uninfluenced by Western paranoia over this movement.

The stretch crunch is not a beginner exercise. A person with weak abs will just jerk on his spine with his hip flexors, even worse than in a conventional crunch. The best tool for stretch crunches is the Swiss ball, an inflatable ball two feet or so in diameter and a $30 price tag. Unlike a rigid pad, the Swiss ball follows the curves of your back and opens up the spaces between vertebrae.

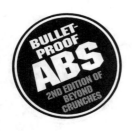

Sit on the ball a bit lower than its top, so your lower back would hit the high point when you lie back. (Fig. 42) Plant your feet slightly wider than your shoulders. You may hook them underneath your couch or have your training partner hold them down, especially if you use additional resistance.

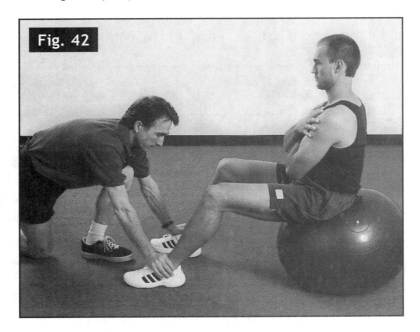

Fig. 42

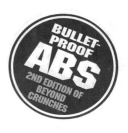

Fold your hands on your chest—eventually with a weight—inhale and <u>wrap yourself around the ball.</u> (Fig. 43)   Do not jam your back in one spot; sort of 'make your spine longer' and wrap it around the deceptively innocent looking ball. You should not experience any discomfort in your lower back if you do the drill right. Make sure to keep your entire midsection tight, your feet secure, and not move too fast—it is hard to stay on the ball!

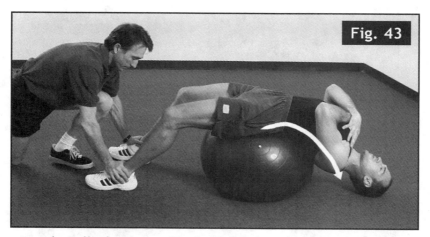

Fig. 43

Incidentally, because of lack of stability the Swiss ball crunch overloads the obliques more than other kinds of situps or crunches.

You will feel it!

At your own risk, try this drill with your feet close together for an even more brutal love handle muscle workout!

When you have reached the bottom exhale with relief and let your spine stretch even longer.

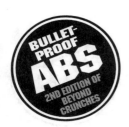

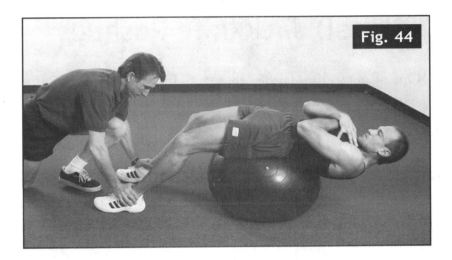

Fig. 44

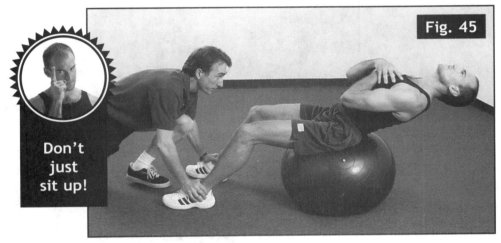

Fig. 45

Don't just sit up!

Inhale, and roll back up, one vertebra at a time starting with your neck. (Fig. 44) Tucking your butt under will help. Do not just sit up (Fig. 45)—curl up!

Once you have reached the top, exhale, inhale, and start over.

Go for it! You will be a hurting unit the morning after!

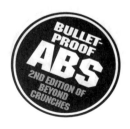

(Wheel) Jackknife Pushups

One of my victims wished there was an especially hot spot in hell for me for having him do wheel jackknives!

The evil wheel (Fig. 46) can be bought for $10 in most sporting goods stores. The package shows off inappropriately smiling ladies. Have them try the wheel my way, and they'll be wailing!

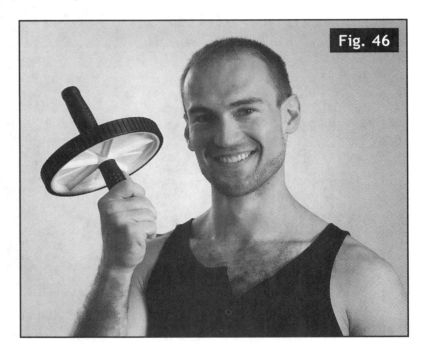

Fig. 46

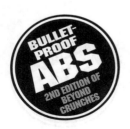

Get down on your knees, the wheel in your hands. Inhale, round your back maximally, tuck your butt and chin in. Your hips should be vertical. (Fig. 47) At no point during the exercise should your butt be sticking out backward, or your back arch! (Fig. 48) Keep your lats, or the armpit muscles, tight to protect your shoulders.

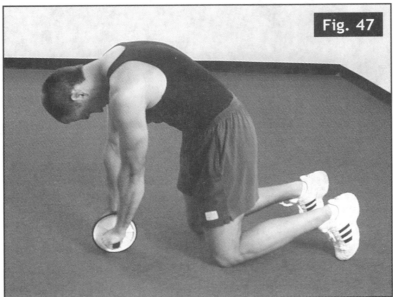
Fig. 47

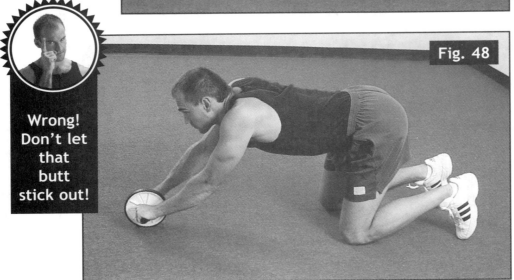
Fig. 48

Wrong! Don't let that butt stick out!

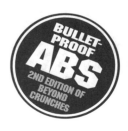

Roll as far as your ability allows you (Fig. 49), and come back up by trying to round your back and simultaneously pulling with your arms. Don't exhale until you reach the top.

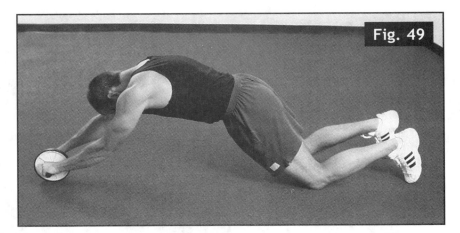

Fig. 49

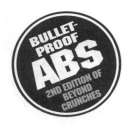

Do not start your descent exaggeratedly slow, you will get tired prematurely, and will crash before reaching the floor. It might be a good idea to have a spotter hold a wide belt under your hips in case you lose control. (Fig. 50) Or you could do the drill in front of a wall, so it stops you before you go too far for your current ability. The stronger you get, the further from the wall you position yourself. I got this tip from Steve Maxwell, the Brazilian Jiu Jitsu Senior World Champion. It is imperative that your back does not arch. Keep it rounded, or at least flat. If you can't and the exercise hurts your lower back, you are not ready for the evil wheel.

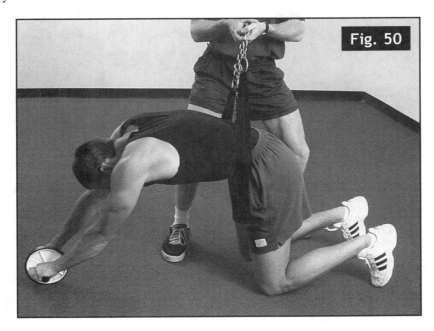

Fig. 50

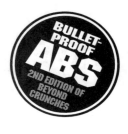

You can do the rep on one breath as suggested above, or you could make your life more miserable (heh-heh!). Once you have reached the wall or the floor—don't try this variation if you do partial reps without a wall! (Fig. 51)—exhale and relax on the floor for a moment.   (Fig. 52) Then inhale, round your back, and come back up to the starting position.

If you can't come up, push up with your arms (Fig. 53A) and continue with your negatives, or the lowering half of the exercise.

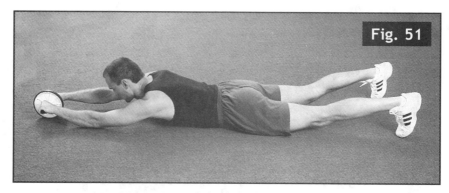

Fig. 51

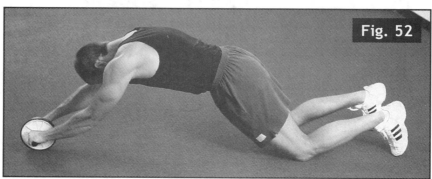

Fig. 52

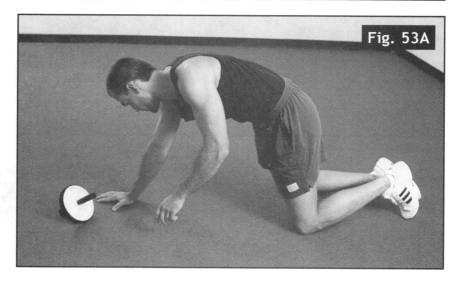

Fig. 53A

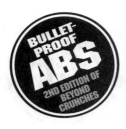

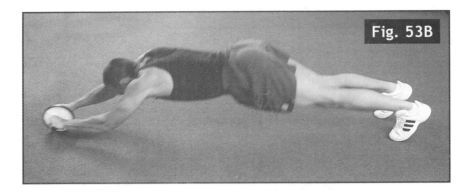

Fig. 53B

Eventually you will be able to reverse the movement, and one day, perhaps, even do the straight-legged version of the exercise where your knees are not touching the floor! (Fig. 53B) While most college jocks would be hard pressed to do one repetition in this manner, Russian health guru Anatoly Kashpirovsky, M.D. cranks out twenty consecutive reps, no problemo!

If you do not have the wheel, you can roll a barbell (Fig. 54).

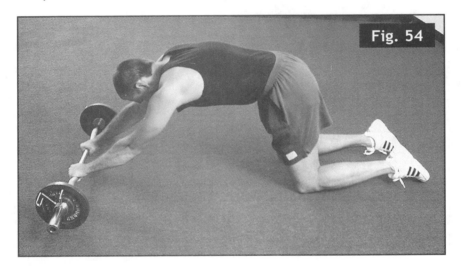

Fig. 54

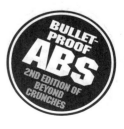

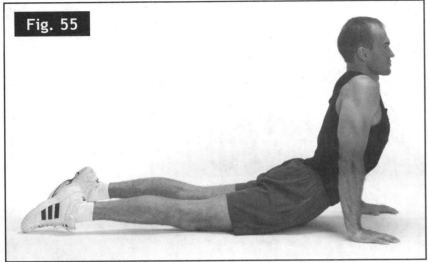

Fig. 55

Another great alternative was proposed in a Russian gymnastics textbook edited by L. P. Orlov in 1952. Assume the pushup position (Fig. 55) with your toes pointed and rested on some low friction surface, e.g. socks on hardwood. Inhale and pull your knees (Fig. 56) forward with your abs, shoulder, and arms (Fig. 57), while keeping most of your weight on your arms. If your toes hurt, relax for a second, and return to the starting position.

Fig. 56

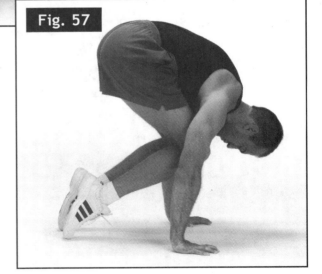

Fig. 57

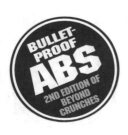

Soviet gymnastics specialist from the Stalin era, S. B. Yananis was big on various pushups for abdominal development. He explained that the abs get a workout by preventing the sagging of the pelvis. I took it to heart and abused the recruits in *Spetsnaz*, the Soviet Special Operations, with brutal jackknife pushups. (Fig. 58)

Stretch out on your stomach, arms overhead, inhale, tuck your butt under, and push up with your hands and feet. 'Keep your armpits tight'. Pause on the top for a count of three, holding your breath and making sure that your back is flat or rounded.

Lower yourself, exhale, and relax for a second before doing another rep. If you cannot keep your back properly aligned and/or experience back discomfort, do an easier version of the jackknife pushups.

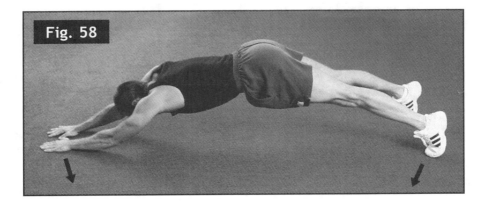

Fig. 58

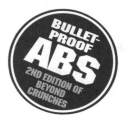

The difficulty of the exercise can be adjusted by changing your leverage: doing it on your knees is easier than on your toes (Fig. 59); resting on your elbows is easier than on your hands (Fig. 60), especially if you move them closer to your body. (Fig. 61) Or combine the two. (Fig. 62) Yananis' pet variation was placing two hands atop each other and resting the head on them. (Fig. 63)

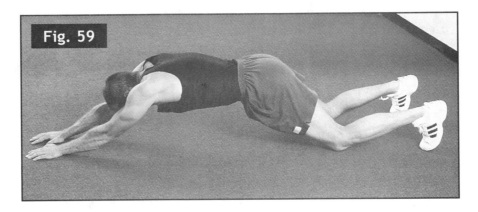

Fig. 59

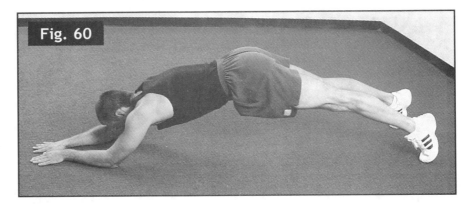

Fig. 60

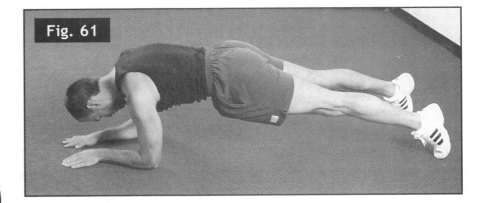

Fig. 61

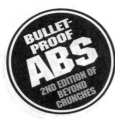

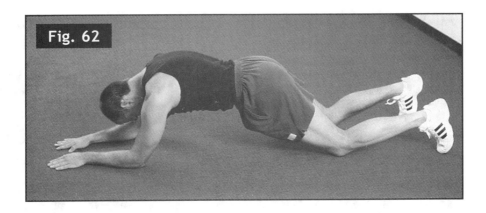

Fig. 62

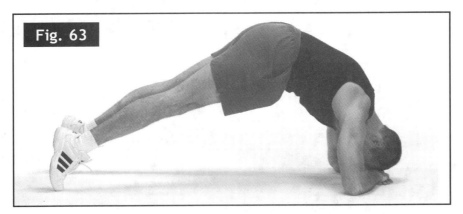

Fig. 63

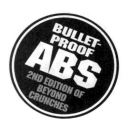

Advanced people can try one arm jackknife pushups (Fig. 64), or the *Spetsnaz* special, the one arm-one leg jackknife! (Fig. 65)

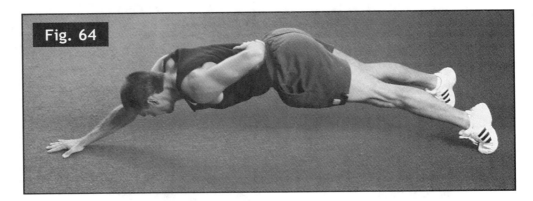

Fig. 64

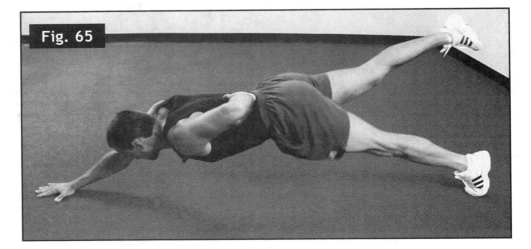

Fig. 65

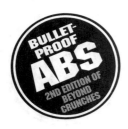

Various pushup drills from Yananis' arsenal, include lifting your legs and arms in different combinations and in different directions. (Fig. 66, 67, 68) A three second hold is considered a rep.

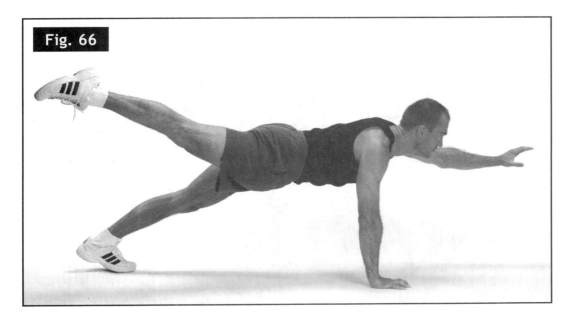

Fig. 66

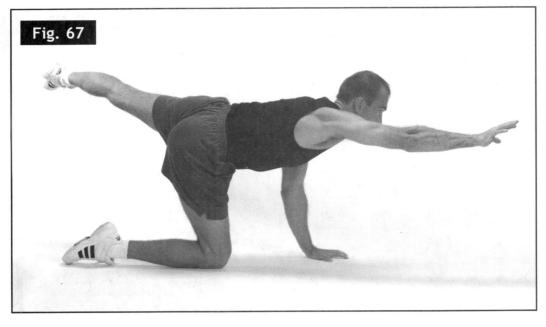

Fig. 67

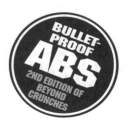

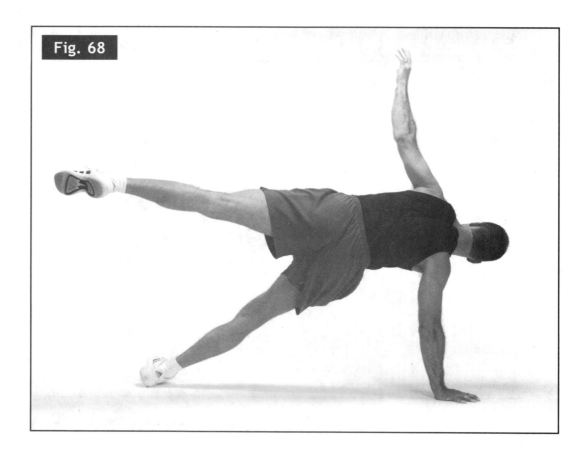

Fig. 68

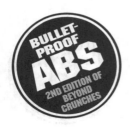

The Russian scientist also recommended hand walking from a crouched position (Fig. 68A, B, C) to the extended position, according to your ability and back—that is one set. East German strength training experts Drs. Jürgen Hartmann and Harold Tünnemannoffered their own evil modification: assume a pushup position (Fig. 69A, B), then walk back as far as your strength allow, and forward to the starting point.   The drill is easier if your hands are elevated above the floor; this offers an opportunity to fine tune the load to your level of conditioning.

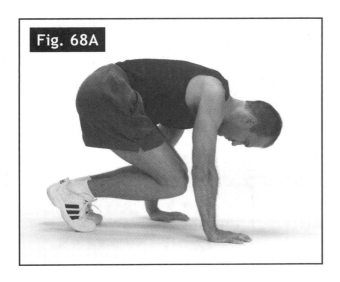

Fig. 68A

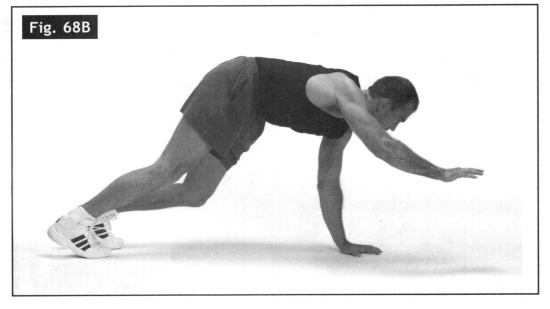

Fig. 68B

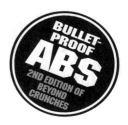

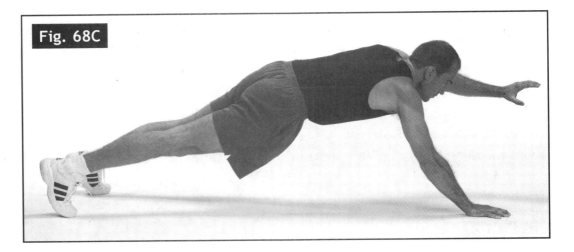

Fig. 68C

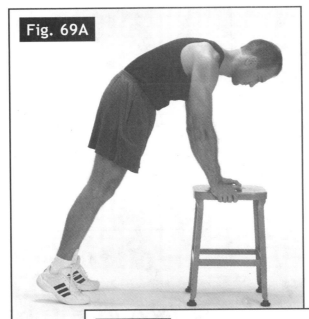

Fig. 69A

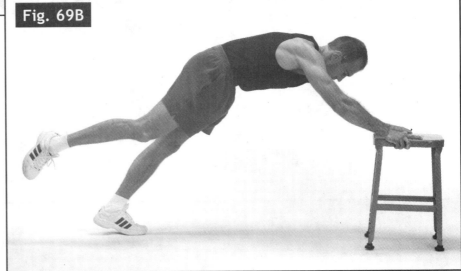

Fig. 69B

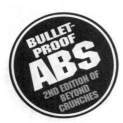

The Dragon Flag

This drill was a favorite of Bruce Lee, a martial arts movie star who possessed what may have been the most ripped abs of all time. Lee called it 'the flag'. Since 'the flag' is a position from gymnastics, I renamed Bruce Lee's exercise to avoid confusion. Let it be called the 'Dragon Flag' in honor of the late Mr. Lee who was nicknamed 'the Little Dragon'.

Do not even dream of trying this very advanced exercise until you can do a wheel jackknife the hard way! Even then it is a good idea to have a spotter in the beginning.

Lie down on an exercise bench holding on to its uprights behind your head. The dragon flag is so severe, it is best to start by cheating your way up and do negatives, or just the lowering half of the drill. Flatten your back, and bring your knees towards your chest while pulling on the bench or its uprights. (Fig. 70)

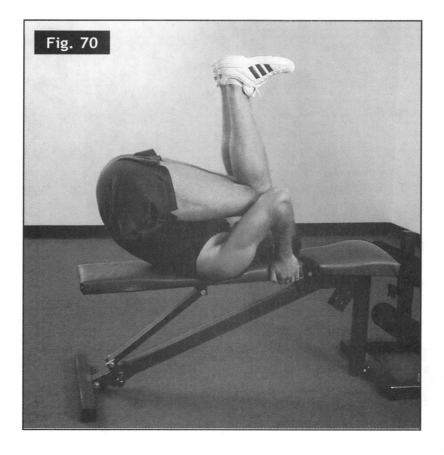

Fig. 70

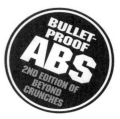

Inhale and extend your body upward, pointing with your toes towards the ceiling and pulling hard with your arms. (Fig. 71) It helps to imagine that you are trying to elongate your spine. Keep your weight on your shoulder blades; do not roll on your neck!

Catch a quick breath, and tighten your abs by tucking in your pelvis.   This is the same move as flattening your back on the floor in the Russian Ballet Leg Thrust. You will not be able to maintain a perfectly flat back throughout this superhuman drill, but try anyway! You can get away with a slight arch as long as it does not hurt your back. Keep your abs locked tight and squeeze your butt hard, silly as it sounds. Tense your lats or 'armpit muscles' as well.

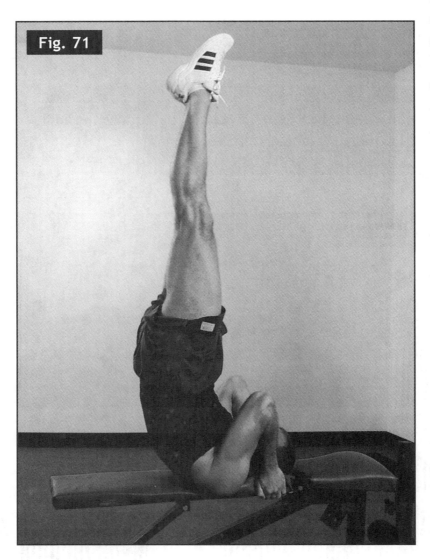

Fig. 71

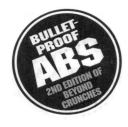

Holding your breath and pulling hard with your arms slowly lower yourself to the bench. Keep your body and legs stretched out. (Fig. 72) Do not jackknife at the hips! (Fig. 73) Pinching an imaginary coin with your buttocks will help.

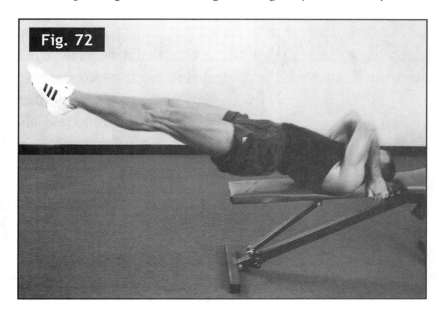

Fig. 72

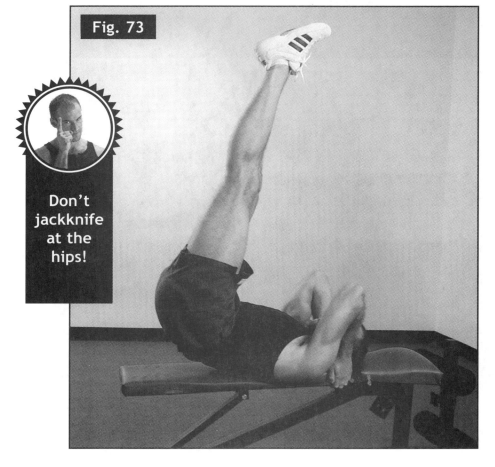

Fig. 73

Don't jackknife at the hips!

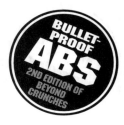

Let out the air with the tension after your feet touch the floor, take a breath, and start all over by cheating your way to the top. When you get good at negatives, do not relax or breathe on the bottom but head back up the same way you came down.

Performing the dragon flag with a Swiss ball (Fig. 74) or a book between your ankles will add another painful touch to this already advanced and somewhat dangerous drill.

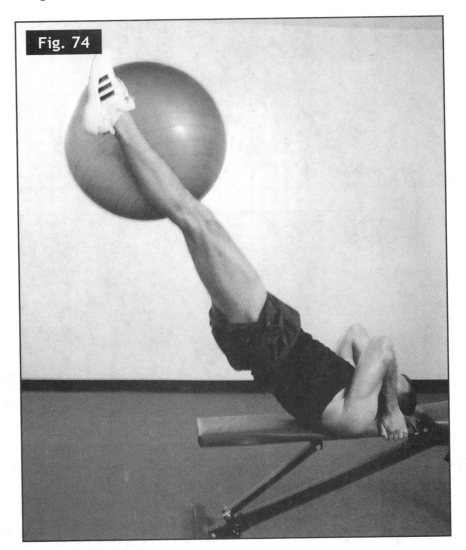

Fig. 74

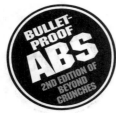

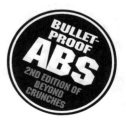

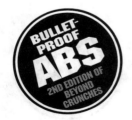

Part III
How to Brutalize the Obliques and Save Your Spine

The obliques are very important to athletes and fitness freaks alike. Strong, well toned obliques make one's waist look trimmer and are critical to performance.

The obliques are the muscles underneath the love handles. Like the abs, they run from your rib cage to your pelvis, but at an angle. The external obliques are aligned in the direction your fingers point when you put your hands in your pockets; the internals run perpendicular to them.

The obliques perform a number of functions when used in different combinations. They laterally flex the spine, as in a side bend, rotate the spine, or help the abs with forward spine flexion.

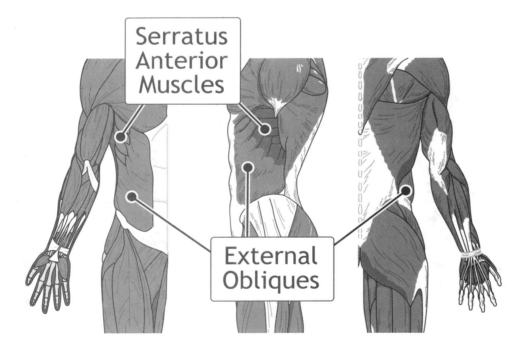

Serratus Anterior Muscles

External Obliques

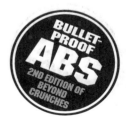

Spine stabilization, as in carrying heavy loads on your shoulders, is another important function of your obliques. The stronger your muscular corset is, the less the wear and tear on your spine.

The few people who train their obliques either do broomstick twists and crunches with a twist—worthless because of the minimal muscular tension they generate—or dangerous twisting situps.

Torsion, simultaneous bending and twisting of the spine, chews up the intervertebral disks.

Once I hurt my back twisting as I bent over holding a 45-pound plate. I was unloading a barbell with many such plates after heavy—and pain free—squats. The moral of the story: a torqued spine is much more vulnerable to an injury than a straight one. Never bend and twist at the same time.

Now, effective training.

Vertebrae (Spinal Bone)

Intervertebral Disk (spongy shock absorber)

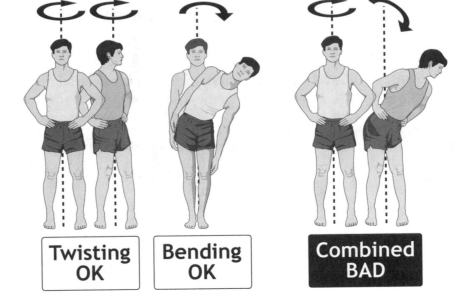

Twisting OK

Bending OK

Combined BAD

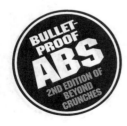

The Full Contact Twist

This unique drill develops an exceptionally tight waist line, and has several martial arts applications.

If you believe that a big bench is the key to punching power, think again. A study performed by Yuri Verkhoshanky and his colleagues—the year the Soviet Empire collapsed—determined that a good boxer's punch derives less than a quarter of its knockout power from the shoulder and arm! Russian research confirmed what martial artists had known for centuries: your striking force is seated in your hips and waist.

The best exercise for transferring the hip power into the shoulder, with a high interest yield, is the Full Contact Twist. This exercise was originally developed in the Soviet Union for shot put conditioning.

The then-nameless twist came to kickboxers' attention when a famous Russian shot putter failed to talk his way out of a mugging. This mild mannered man got annoyed when one of the attackers cut him with a blade. He ruptured the punk's spleen with a single punch.

Igor Sukhotsky, M.Sc., formerly a nationally ranked weightlifter and an eccentric sports scientist who took up full contact karate at the age of fort-five, popularized the twist among Russian fighters. This renaissance man noticed that the twist not only had increased his striking power, but also had toughened his midsection against blows by toning it up. Sukhotsky was so impressed with the Full Contact Twist, that he added it to his super abbreviated strength training routine which consisted of only four exercises: squats, bench presses, deadlifts, and good mornings.

Load a barbell on one side and stick the other end in the corner. A hundred pound plate on the end of the bar is a very reasonable goal for a serious athlete, but be sensible and start with a Barbie plate or an empty bar.

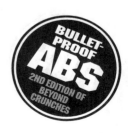

Use a folded towel or some other padding to protect the wall. (Fig. 75) Pick up the loaded end of the bar, using your legs (Fig. 76), rather than your back, and hold it in front of you with your fingers interlocked. The bar should be at approximately 45 degrees from the floor, although you may have to adjust the angle to suit your height and leverage.

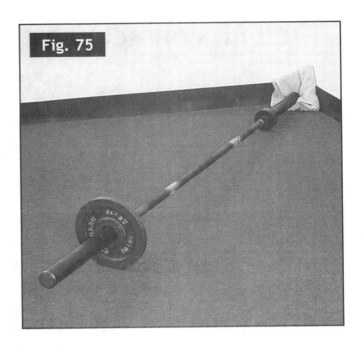

Fig. 75

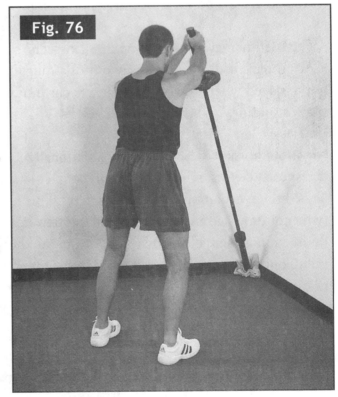

Fig. 76

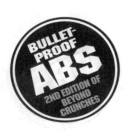

Keep your back and arms straight, your knees bent. If you have a hard time keeping your elbows locked, concentrate on flexing your triceps. Remaining upright, inhale and turn the weight to one side while holding your breath. Don't lean with the bar (Fig. 77), or away from the bar. (Fig. 78)

Pivot on your toes at the same time to avoid shearing forces on your knees. (Fig. 79A) Make sure to wear shoes that do not catch on the surface where you are exercising. No shoes is dandy too.

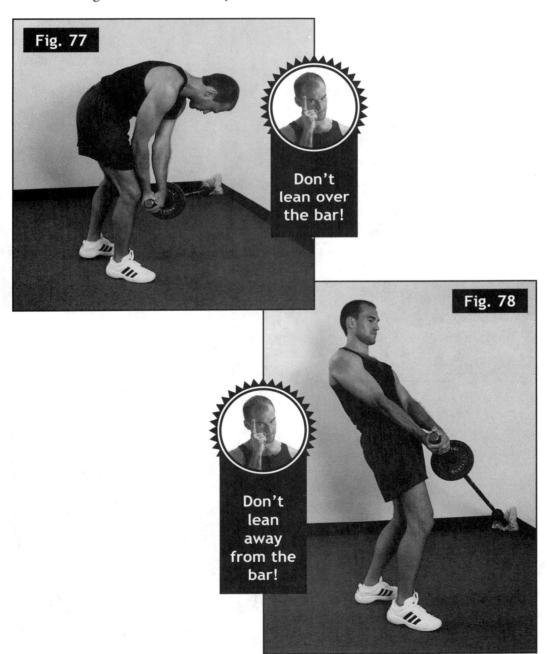

Fig. 77

Don't lean over the bar!

Fig. 78

Don't lean away from the bar!

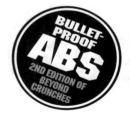

Reverse the movement by tightening up your midsection and rotating your hips. (Fig. 79B) Do not lift with your arms and shoulders. Do not exhale until you reach the top of the lift.

Control the weight at all times. Repeat the exercise in the opposite direction. That was one rep.

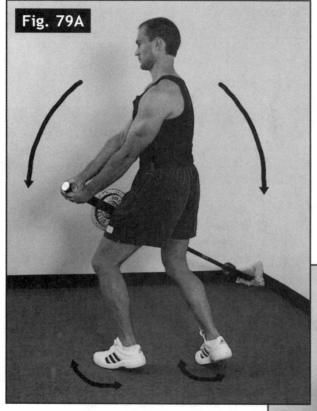

Fig. 79A

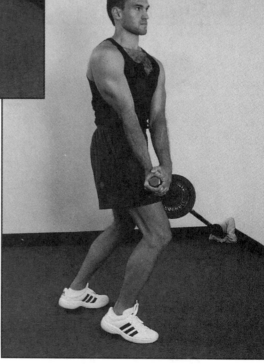

Fig. 79B

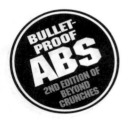

The Saxon Side Bend

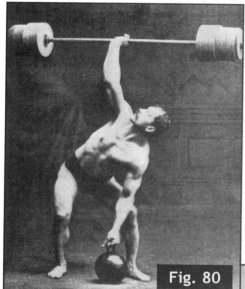

Fig. 80

This deceptively easy looking move was a favorite of old time German strong man Arthur Saxon. He was famous for his exceptional strength and a sinewy, wiry physique (Fig. 80).

Grab two light dumbbells or barbell plates and lift them overhead. (Fig. 81) Don't make do with only one weight—it will make the exercise easier and less effective.

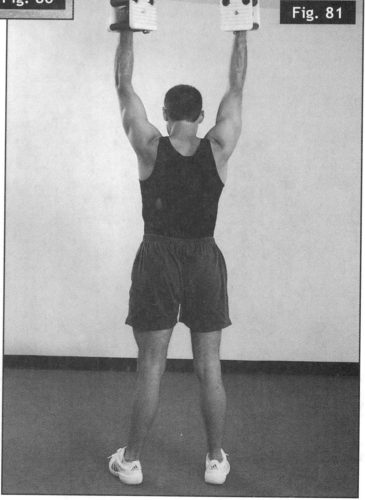

Fig. 81

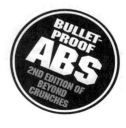

Inhale, elongate your spine, and slowly bend strictly sideways. (Fig. 82) You will find that you cannot go very deep and will be tempted to twist, but don't!—it does your back no good. Don't lean back either for the same reason. Pause for a moment in the lowest position while keeping your entire midsection tight, squeeze your butt, and head back. This glute contraction will make it a lot easier to get the weights moving from this awkward position without twisting.

Exhale when you are upright, inhale again, and bend to the opposite side. Keep the dumbbells the same distance apart throughout the set—that is the hard part.

With the Saxon Side Bends you will not only get a great oblique workout, but will train your shoulders and back as well.

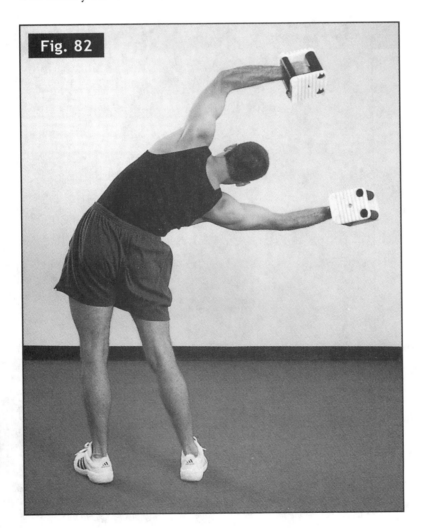

Fig. 82

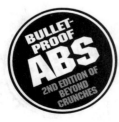

The Suitcase Style One-Arm Deadlift

This is really a full body exercise with an effect you must experience to believe. The day after you try it you will feel like you have been run over by a semi! You will especially feel your obliques, glutes, upper and lower back, thighs… Name a muscle, you will feel it! The One-Arm Deadlifts also strengthen the *quadrotus lumborum*, deep muscles on the sides of the lower spine, important for back health and difficult to develop.

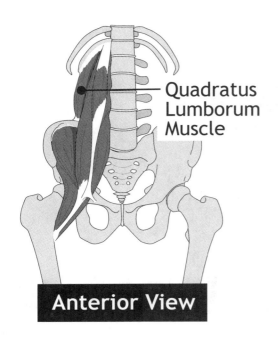

Quadratus Lumborum Muscle

Anterior View

A barbell, rather than a dumbbell is used for two reasons. First, the former takes a very dedicated effort to drop on your foot. And second, a long bar will develop spectacular grip. You will be humbled at how difficult it is to control it and how hard you will have to squeeze it. Once you cannot hold onto the weight your body can still lift, you may try the so called 'hook grip' employed by weightlifters, or wrap the first knuckle of your thumb with your index and middle fingers. Still make a point of squeezing the bar. Be careful to ease into the hook grip, your thumbs will thank you for it. But no matter what you do, don't be pathetic and resort to wrist straps!

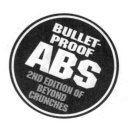

If a 45 pound Olympic bar is too heavy for you to start with, or your grip is too weak to control such a long barbell, try a 15 pound 'EZ' curl bar for starters. (Fig. 83)

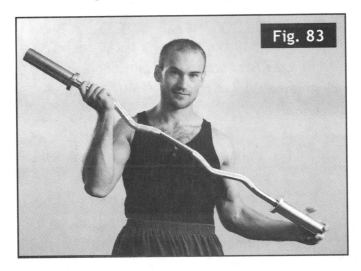

Fig. 83

Stand on one side of a loaded barbell, almost brushing it with your calf. Your toes should be pointed forward and your feet should be a little closer together than your shoulders. The center of the bar should be even with the middle of your feet. Look out, inhale and 'grow' taller by elongating your spine as your rib cage expands. (Fig. 84)

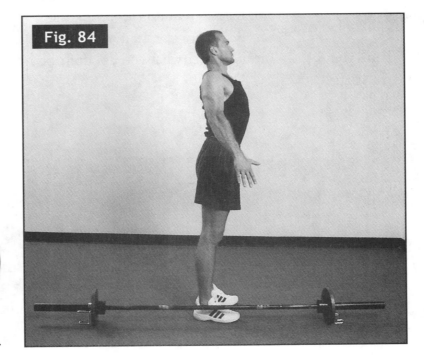

Fig. 84

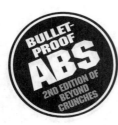

Sit back on your heels, sticking your butt out and keeping your weight on your heels. (Fig. 85)

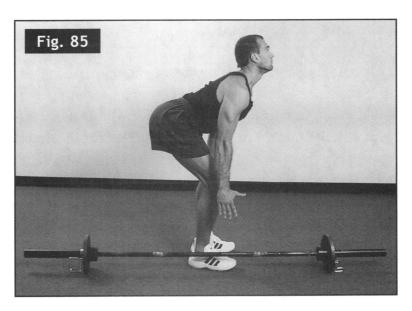

Fig. 85

Don't just go down. (Fig. 86) This shifts your weight forward on your toes making it impossible to use the strong hip muscles and putting unhealthy stress on your knees.

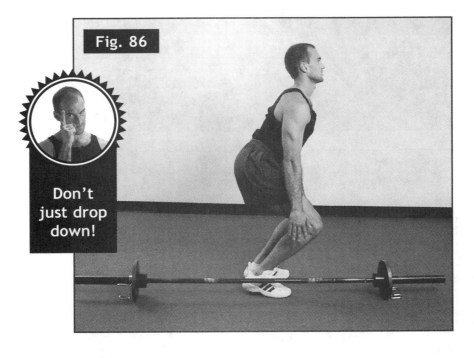

Fig. 86

Don't just drop down!

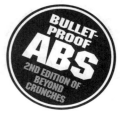

Grab the bar very hard—crush it!—and push the floor away. That's right, don't pull on the bar, just push the floor away, as in a leg press. This is a neat visualization Olympic weightlifters use—to learn how to lift with their legs, rather than backs and arms.

Make sure that your arm is straight and tense when you start the lift, flex your triceps. Yanking on the barbell or curling does not help to lift much iron and could injure your arm or back. Consider the analogy of starting towing a car with a slack cable. Keep your back straight for the duration of the drill.

This exercise is not a side bend, and not a twist! Your body should raise evenly. (Fig. 87) It helps your balance to imagine that you lift a suitcase in each hand.(Fig. 88)

Semi-exhale as you reach the top. (Fig. 88) Do not lean back or sideways with the weight.

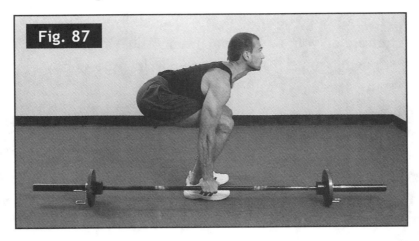

Fig. 87

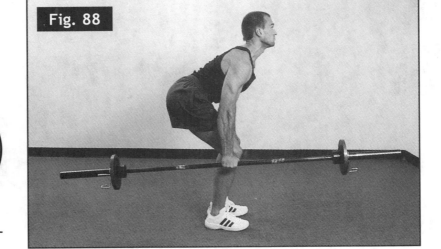

Fig. 88

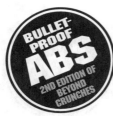

Semi-exhale as you reach the top. (Fig. 89) Do not lean back or sideways with the weight.

Inhale and sit back. Don't think of lowering the bar. It will make your descent crooked and use too much back. Just sit back. The weight will take care of itself.

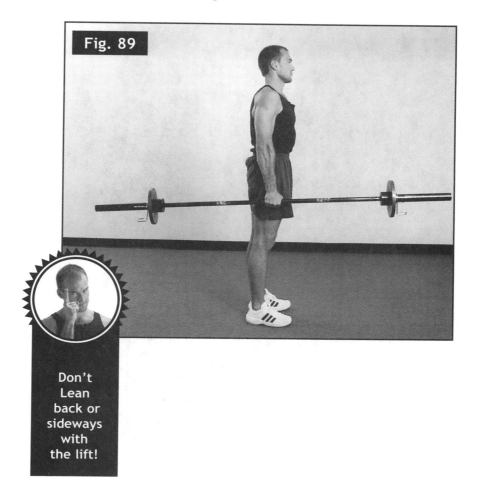

Fig. 89

Don't
Lean
back or
sideways
with
the lift!

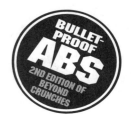

It is hard to set the bar down in exactly the same spot as you had picked it up. (Fig. 90) The unintelligent piece of metal tends to land an inch or two in front of where it should be. Keep that in mind and make the necessary correction. Set it down a little further back than you should.

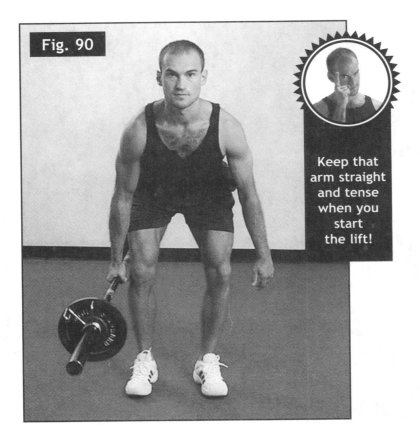

Fig. 90

Keep that arm straight and tense when you start the lift!

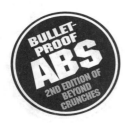

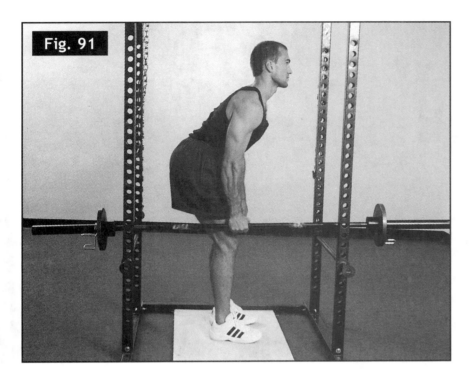

Fig. 91

People with long torsos and short arms usually have difficulty picking up a weight off the floor in good form and should do most of their deadlifting in a power rack or off some sturdy blocks. (Fig. 91) Come to think of it, so do most Comrades unfamiliar with the One-Arm Deadlift.

The coolest way to incorporate power rack deadlifts in your schedule is *neurological carryover*. Start with the bar at your knee level and lower it an inch or so every third workout. If the space between the pin holes in your rack is more then two inches, stand on plywood to make smaller jumps. In the olden days lifters would dig a hole in the ground and deadlift while standing in it. They would lengthen the movement by adding an inch of dirt every few workouts. Eventually the hole would fill up and the strongman would pull a full deadlift with a weight he used to be able to budge only a few inches!

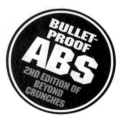

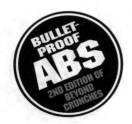

Part IV

How to Boost Yourself from Wannabe to Champion with Power Breathing

Warning! Many American physicians believe that holding your breath during exercise could be hazardous to your health. If you have a heart problem, high blood pressure, or other health concerns, consult your physician before attempting any of the breathing patterns described in this book!

While sports scientists from the former Soviet Union emphasize special exercises for the respiratory muscles and recommend state of the art breathing patterns to be employed during exertion, all the Western breathing wisdom can be summed up in "inhale as you go down, exhale as you go up". This advice got old around the days of the Boston Tea Party.

There are two types of exhalation which are worlds apart: *active* and *passive*. A pagan Russian berserker's war scream or the grunt of a strongman bending a horse shoe are examples of the former. The sigh of relief you give out after a successful job interview is a latter. The profoundly different effects these breathing patterns have on your physical performance are known in Russia as the *pneumo-muscular reflex*. This neurological phenomenon can be compared to the amplifier of your stereo where your brain is the CD player and your muscles are the speakers. Special *baroreceptors* in your abdominal and thoracic cavities register the internal pressure and adjust your muscular tension like the volume control knob. The higher is this pressure, the greater your strength and vice versa.

The skill of picking the breathing pattern appropriate for the task at hand separates the great athlete from the also-ran. When I teach martial artists to do splits, I show them how to rid their muscles of tension with a 'let go' passive exhalation. It should be obvious that an attempt to duplicate this breathing pattern under heavy metal dooms you for weakness and injuries. By the same token, constricting your respiratory muscles as if you are deadlifting five wheels during a stretch will only lead to ripped muscles and the flexibility of a cadaver.

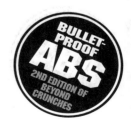

Martial artists have possessed the knowledge of the pneumo-muscular reflex for centuries. They expressed it as 'matching the breath with the force'. A karate master synchronizing a board splintering strike with a blood curdling "K-i-a-i!" does exactly that. Sudden squeezing of the air by a powerful contraction of the respiratory muscles and the abdominals peaks the internal pressure at the moment of the impact. This maneuver dramatically increases the muscular tension, or force, for a fraction of a second. By the same token, fighters know that once the power breath is out, you are there for the taking and you had better get out of the way!

How does all this relate to ab training? First, use <u>a breathing pattern that maximizes the intra-abdominal pressure: groan, scream, hiss, or just plain hold your breath. Second, maintain high IAP until the end of the rep or half rep. Do not expel all of your air too soon, or you will lose tightness and strength.</u> A repetition of a strength drill lasts a lot longer than a punch. Try to kiai your way out of a four hundred pound bench press, and the bar will collapse your sternum as surely as a karate chop! As you exhale forcefully, you will amplify your strength for a moment—only to become weak as a kitten once your bad breath is out. Run out of air too soon during a wheel jackknife—and your chiropractor might upgrade his Mercedes to this year's model.

Which power breathing technique should you chose? Any of the above will do, as long as you have cleared it with your doctor. A 1977 Soviet study by Vorobyev determined that both holding one's breath and groaning increase strength. Screaming is not bad either. According to the 1961 study by Ikai and Steinhaus, subjects who shouted during exertion got a respectable 12.2% strength boost!

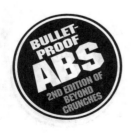

Bending the Fire

You will be able to squeeze even more juice out of either power breathing pattern if you practice the following drill recommended by Prof. Vladimir Zatsiorsky, a renegade Russian strength authority. This exercise is sometimes called in the martial arts circles 'Bending the Fire' because that is what your breath would do to the flame of a candle if you had one in front of you.

Take a normal breath—former weightlifting world champion Russian Prof. Arkady Vorobyev recommends 75% of your maximal air intake for peak strength performance —and flex your abs. At the same time contract your rectal sphincter as if you are trying to stop yourself from going to the bathroom. This bizarre maneuver from Iron Shirt Chi Kung further increases the inside pressure and amplifies your strength. The anal lock also acts as an insurance against hemorrhoids. Gym rats and couch potatoes alike tend to let their intestines go when they strain. Such a constipated style of strength training could lead to health problems and offers no performance advantage. Always pull up the muscles of the pelvic floor when you lift!

Expel the air forcefully in three to five seconds while keeping you glottis closed and your butt pulled in. It helps if you synchronize the expiration with arm movement. (Fig. 92-96) Push forward or downward to peak the contraction of the midsection musculature. The Force is with you if you sound like Darth Vader.

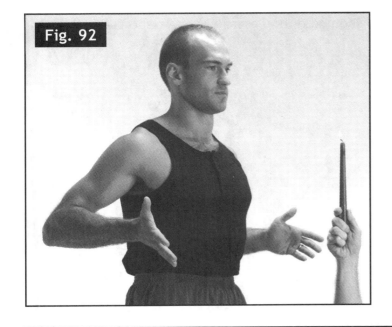

Fig. 92

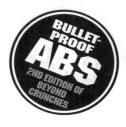

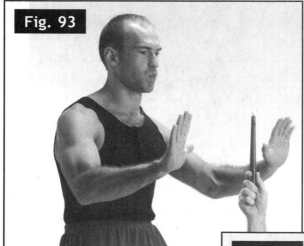

Fig. 93

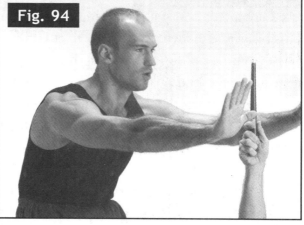

Fig. 94

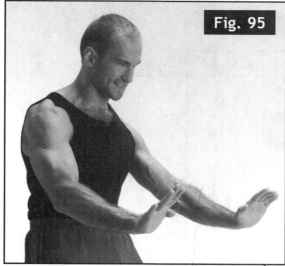

Fig. 95

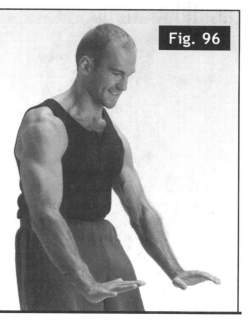

Fig. 96

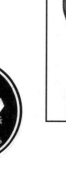

The Second Focus

To add an extra kick to the already awesome Bending the Fire, once you have expelled almost all of your air, blast out the rest with an explosive grunt! (Fig. 99) This 'Second Focus' exercise is the cornerstone of *tameshiwari,* the martial arts practice of breaking boards, bricks, etc.

Totally relax between reps. Zatsiorsky recommends ten to fifteen contractions per set, three to four sets spread throughout the day, every day. You know me, I would double the sets and halve the reps (buy my book *Power to the People!* if you want to know why).

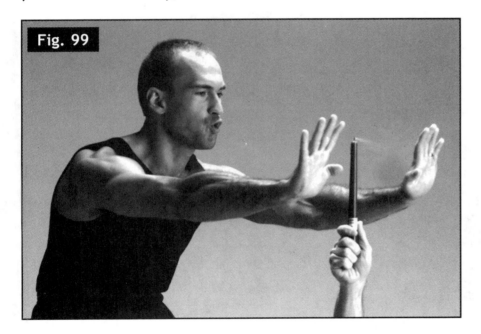

Fig. 99

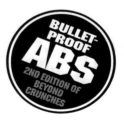

The below drill is more than just breathing practice; it is a powerful strengthener of all the midsection muscles. (Fig. 97, 98) Vladimir Zatsiorsky cites a double-blind study that showed this type of exercise to be superior to any other!

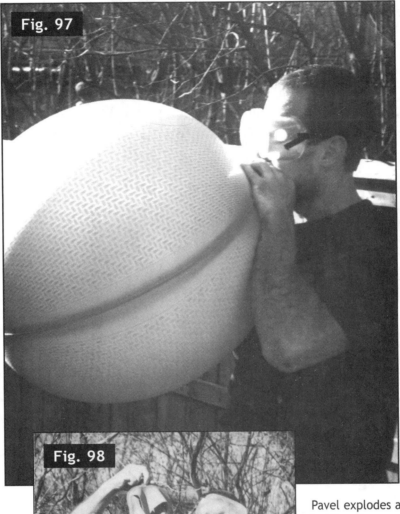

Fig. 97

Fig. 98

Pavel explodes a water bottle using a variation of *Bending the Fire* breathing

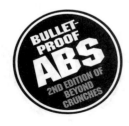

The Elbow Strike Second Focus

If you combine the Second Focus with an elbow strike, you will not believe the intensity of the contraction of your side muscles, the obliques and serratus anterior. Of course, this will translate into, as the Irish say, "more power to your elbow", and a smaller, ripped to shreds, waist line!

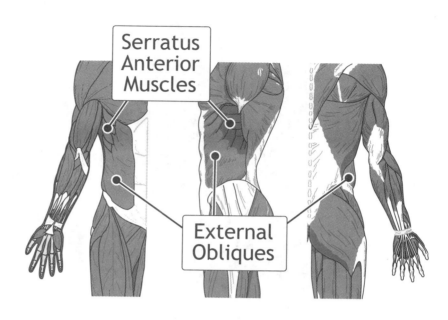

Serratus Anterior Muscles

External Obliques

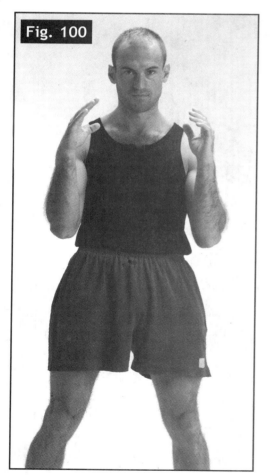

Fig. 100

Assume the on-guard position. (Fig. 100)

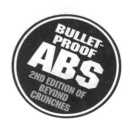

BULLET-PROOF ABS
2ND EDITION OF BEYOND CRUNCHES

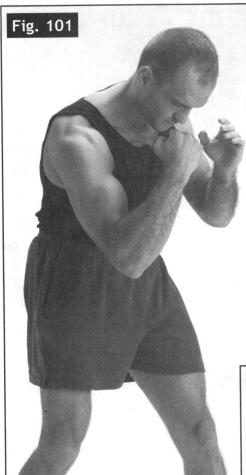

Fig. 101

Start the Bending the Fire sequence imagining that you are about to break a brick positioned in front of you at your hip level. (Fig. 101) Perform the Second Focus as your elbow reaches the virtual brick (Fig. 102). Do not try to twist! (Fig. 103) While the limited rotation of the efficient strike delivers power, conscious twisting will do more damage to your back than good for your midriff.

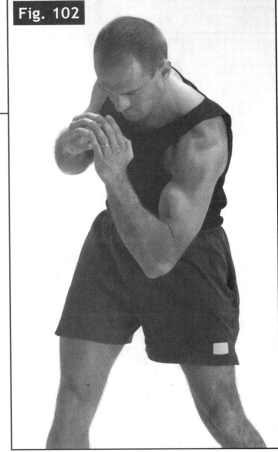

Fig. 102

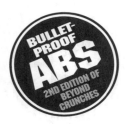

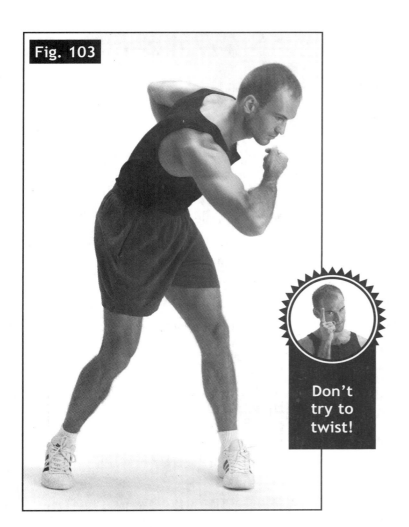

Fig. 103

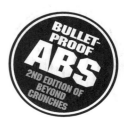

Don't try to twist!

The Second Focus/Ab Pavelizer™ Negative Sequence

This move would have been practiced in the GULAG had it been invented in Stalin's days! Assume the seated, top position on your Ab Pavelizer™ and perform the Second Focus drill.

Once you have expelled all the air and all the muscles between your ribcage and your pelvis went into a lethal cramp—hold that contraction and lower yourself to the ground without inhaling! Once you are down you may wish to get back up in the normal fashion, or just get up with the help of your arms. If you are really tough, perform the Bending the Fire drill as you are doing the Janda situp and put an exclamation mark with the Second Focus when you have reached the sitting position. (Fig. 104-106)

You can do the same sequence with the elbow strike. Keep your knees apart and strike a virtual target with your elbow. Again, twist as you strike, do not twist to strike! The martial move naturally rotates your shoulder without wrenching your lower back as dangerous and ineffective twisting situps.

If you have used the right elbow, lower yourself to the ground with most of your weight on the right leg and vice versa. I shall be redundant: do not twist on the way down, just keep your weight shifted on one side!

<u>Warning! Be aware that Bending the Fire and the Second Focus, with or without the negative, are not meant to be employed within the context of the majority of other strength training exercises, abdominal and otherwise!</u> You become vulnerable following the extreme exhalation and most drills do not boast such a nice, safe finishing position as the Ab Pavelizer™ situps.

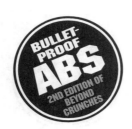

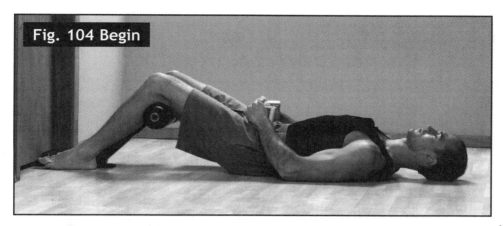

Fig. 104 Begin

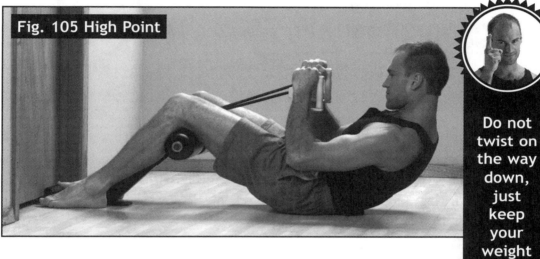

Fig. 105 High Point

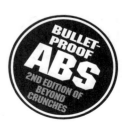

Do not twist on the way down, just keep your weight shifted to one side!

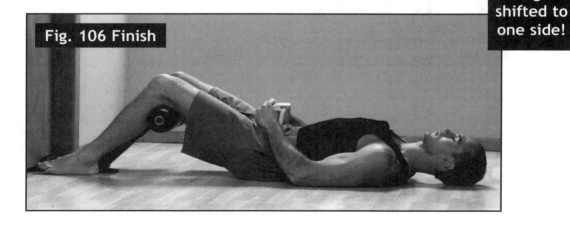

Fig. 106 Finish

The Vacuum

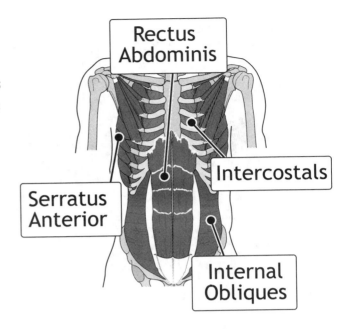

Rectus Abdominis

Intercostals

Serratus Anterior

Internal Obliques

In addition to sending ripples through the superficial muscles of the abdominal wall, the above power breathing drill tightens up your *transversus abdominis*, the muscle that supports your viscera. Some Yoga practitioners have strengthened this muscle to the point where you can see their spines in the front when they suck their stomachs in!

This Yoga drill known in the West as 'the vacuum' delivers multiple health benefits, such as defeating constipation, and one cosmetic one: a smaller waist. The Vacuum strengthens your *intercostals* (Fig. 107), the muscles that elevate your ribs, and compliments the effects of the power breathing martial arts exercises.

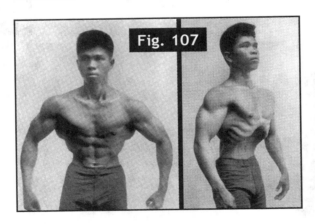

Fig. 107

Simon Javierto demonstrating the phases of isolation of the abdominal muscles. This control is accomplished by complete exhalation of all air from the lungs drawing in the abdominal wall to fill the vacuum (second photo). Then by bending forward and contracting the rectus abdominus (first photo). (Photo from Earle Liederman)

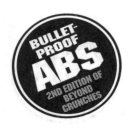

Exhale all your air —with the Second Focus if you wish—and expand your ribcage to the max without inhaling. (new photo 29) The vacuum in your lungs will literally pull your stomach up. Hold the vacuum for a few seconds, and relax.

This drill does not take a lot out of you, so it should be done more frequently than the rest—every day throughout the day. It helps if you develop a pattern, a reminder, for instance do vacuum on every red light, or when waiting for the elevator.

To do a more advanced version of this exercise, get down on your fours. (Fig. 108) You will not only work against the resiliency of your viscera, but also against the gravity.

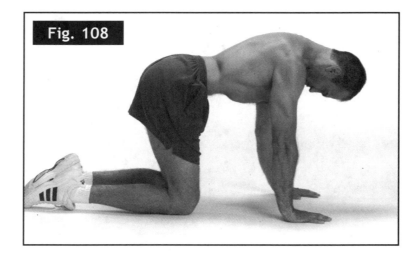

Fig. 108

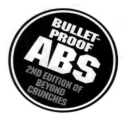

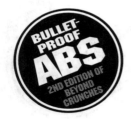

Part V
Questions & Answers

Q: Everybody knows that abs should be 'burned' with high reps and a very light weight. You recommend heavy low rep training. Don't you get it that I don't want to build my abs?! I just want to tone them!

Chill out, Ma'am. 'Everybody' should not have slept through their Physiology 101. The 'burn' you feel from high reps is from lactic acid buildup and does absolutely nothing for toning up your muscles. Tone is residual tension in a relaxed muscle. The logical way to develop it is by tensing the muscle. High tension training is high resistance training.

High repetitions and high resistance are mutually exclusive. Voila!

Now, in order to understand why you will not build up your waist following my program, you have to understand how muscle is built—and then do the opposite.

In cybernetics, the science about control in different, including biological, systems, there is a concept of the black box. A VCR is a black box. You do not know what is inside, yet you get what you want. Pop a tape into the VCR, switch your TV to Channel 3, and the *Star Wars* are back. Only the cause and effect matter.

Nobody knows what happens inside a muscle when it grows bigger. However, we know what buttons to push to get the hypertrophic response. These buttons are tension and fatigue.

Tension is a function of the load—the heavier the weight or the more challenging the exercise, the higher is the tension. At a first glance it makes sense to train with maximal weights.

However, a weight that is too heavy cannot be lifted enough times to induce a high level of fatigue. A light weight lifted to failure will tire your muscles out but the tension will be pathetic. A Catch-22.

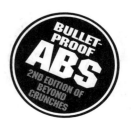

To trigger muscle hypertrophy one has to reach a certain compromise of fatigue and tension, the fatigue/tension threshold. I am simplifying things somewhat, but a weight that you can lift for 30-60 seconds, or around 6-12 times before failure generates enough tension and fatigue to build muscle.

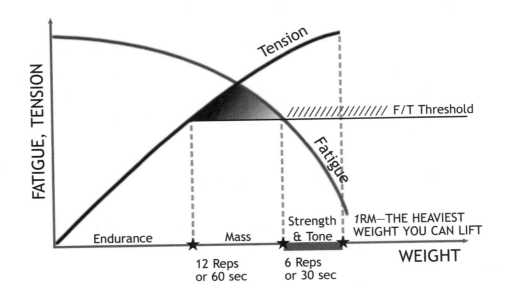

Keep your sets under half a minute, or, even under twenty seconds, cut your reps to five and under. To avoid cumulative fatigue bump up the rest intervals between the sets to—gasp!—three to five minutes, and keep your set total to five and under. You can easily remember this as the '3-5 method': 3-5 sets, 3-5 reps, 3-5 minutes of rest between sets. Such a radical workout will only make you harder and stronger—not bigger.

As for the wimpy high rep stuff, it's not only more than worthless, it can puff you up! Such training, or 'muscle spinning', was popular among California bodybuilders back in the fifties. They were big, weak, and soft.

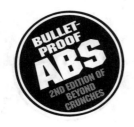

High repetitions develop muscular endurance. In the case of the 15-50 rep range most 'shapers' and 'toners' use, it is anaerobic, or short term, endurance. In this mode your muscles burn glycogen, a form of sugar, for fuel. It is stored, among other places, in the muscles. High rep training depletes your glycogen reserves. To prevent such a critical situation in the future, your body will store more glycogen than before. Now here is the catch. Each molecule of this substance binds with three molecules of water. Jiggle, jiggle! You look like you could cross the Sahara desert without refueling!

Q: I heard that a muscle should be 'confused' by changing my workout constantly. How should I do it?

No matter how well designed your workout is, it is not going to work forever. The physiological Law of Accommodation states that an organism stops adapting to a training stimulus after a period of time, usually four to six weeks. Your body figures, "Hey, it hasn't killed me yet, why bother to adapt?" At this point a change in the program is called for. The change can be quantitative like increasing the number of sets or cycling the workload in a manner described in my book *Power to the People!: Russian Strength Training Secrets for Every American*, or qualitative, that is replacing the exercises.

The *Bullet-Proof Abs* approach to refreshing your workout is straightforward: pick one or two drills from this book, focus on them for a month or so, then switch to something else. It is a good idea to do Janda situps every other rotation.

Do not fall for 'muscle confusion' or changing your exercises every workout. Adaptation to constantly changing stimuli is impossible by definition. A shotgun mix of exercises confuses the organism by constantly changing demands instead of shocking it into specific adaptation. Overhauling your workout too often is just as bad as doing the same old thing for too long. It is OK though to vary your sets, reps, and rest intervals every session. Be careful to stay more or less within the 3-5 limits if you do not want to bulk up.

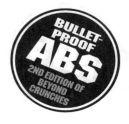

Q: Are 'negatives' good for toning the abs?

Excellent!

'Negatives', or the lowering half of an exercise, generate up to 1.3 times more muscular tension than 'positives', or the lifting half.

Look at the force-velocity curve. There is an inverse relationship between the force of the contraction and its velocity. The slower the contraction, the higher is the force (tension). When the speed of contraction is negative, the tension is at its highest values.

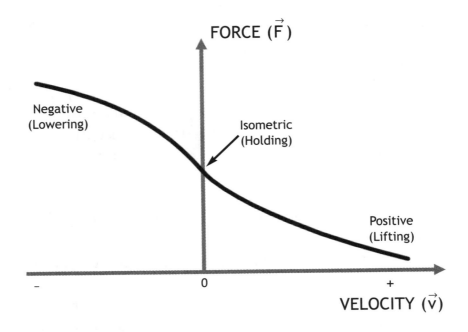

Research suggests that the optimal load for negative training is one that you can lower slowly and halt at will. Don't use a weight that is too heavy and makes you lose muscular tension and fall like a rock!

Not every exercise lends itself to negatives and some drills, e.g. the Saxon Side Bend, require spotters if you choose to employ this training modality. Use your head.

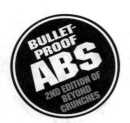

Q: What about isometrics?

If you look at the force-velocity curve one more time, you will see that isometric training, or holding the weight, rather than lifting it, also induces more tension than lifting.

A very effective way of incorporating isometrics into your ab training regimen is the Soviet static-dynamic method. It requires you to pause for three seconds at different stages of an exercise, especially at the hardest spot. Do not hold your breath if you use this technique; breathe shallow while keeping your core tight.

Q: What do you think of super slow training for the abs?

The force-velocity curve says it works. The lower is the velocity, the higher is the tension. Super slow works. But, like everything else, it works best if you switch to something else after a while. A 1975 Russian study by S. I. Lelikov determined that a program which varied the exercise tempo over a period of time was roughly 150% more effective in developing strength than constant super slow training!

Q: Can I develop great definition in my abs with only one set of an exercise?

You might, but I would not bet on it.

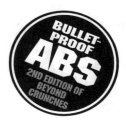

Q: Is your low rep program going to give me a 'six-pack'?

The program was designed to strengthen and harden your abs. If you want a prominent six-pack, the abdominals have to be built to a degree. One way of doing it is to finish your heavy low rep workout with a lighter set of over 20 seconds in duration, or 6-12 reps to failure, assuming an average lifting tempo. You can do the same, or a different, exercise. For example:

1.	Situps:	3x5 @ 35 pounds
2.	Situps:	1x12 @ 10 pounds

1.	Scissor situps:	4x4 @ 25 pounds
2.	Ab Pavelizer™ situps:	1x10 @ bodyweight only

Or you could simply do more sets, e.g. 10x5, and compress the rest intervals between them to 1-3 min.

Q: Can I train my abs every day?

Soviet research demonstrated that athletes who increase the number of their weekly workouts while keeping their training volume—or the total number of repetitions—constant, immediately show a significant strength increase. If you do 5x5 once a week, 1x5 five times a week will be more effective. My dad Vladimir Tsatsouline has recently worked up to seventeen consecutive pullups by doing this exercise every morning. He could not do that many at any point of his thirty-two-year service in the Soviet Army.

Yet I am not pushing for daily training or multiple daily workouts because it is not practical for most people. You can get great results training three times a week. If you choose to train more often, spread the sets you have been doing over more workouts. Later, when you can comfortably handle the load, you might want to add sets.

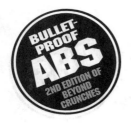

Another option is to pick an exercise you can do anywhere, for example the Russian ballet leg thrust or the jackknife pushup, and do a set of up to five reps here and there throughout the day. It is imperative that you try to avoid fatigue when following this method! Your last set of the day should feel almost as fresh as the first one.

Q: I don't have health club membership and can't do the one arm deadlift and the full contact twist. Any suggestions?

Buy a 300 pound Olympic weight set. It sells in most sporting goods stores for around $150, including the bar.

Q: Can I do twists on a Nautilus machine instead of the full contact twist?

I wouldn't.

Unlike the abs, the obliques do not need to be isolated for maximal training effect. Remember the *Law of Irradiation*. A contraction of a muscle amplifies the contraction of the adjacent muscles. What was a liability in ab training is an asset in oblique training. The tension in the hips and abs will enable you to lift more weight and better overload you obliques.

Also, the full contact twist teaches athletes to integrate their hip, midsection, and upper body efforts into a lethal punch or other sport skill.

Q: Do I have to do separate exercises for my abs and my obliques?

If you wish. Either way you work the entire midsection, just with a different emphasis.

Q: Many muscle magazines recommend doing ab exercises before lifting weights. Do you think it is a good idea?

Definitely not. These muscles stabilize the spine under heavy loads, and pre-exhausting them could lead to back injuries later in your workout.

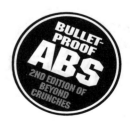

Q: What kind of warmup and stretching exercises do I need to do before training my abs?

None, with the rare exception of the back stretch described in the chapter about the Ab Pavelizer™.

I have explained in great detail why warming up is a waste of time in my stretching book. You can find the order information at the end of this volume.

If you have hyperlordosis, or an exaggerated arch in your lower back, you need to stretch your hip flexors. A couple of state of the art hip flexor stretches are covered in my new stretching book. Remember to clear the stretches with your doctor if you intend to do them to correct a medical condition.

Q: You are saying crunches do not work. It doesn't make any sense. My aerobic instructor swears this is all she does for her abs—and she looks fantastic!

Do you believe that Cindy Crawford looks like Cindy Crawford because of the exercises she demonstrates on her tapes, or because she was born Cindy Crawford?

Business heavyweight Robert Ringer once said that successful people often do not know what really got them to the top. Translation: you can rely on no authority but hard scientific facts and common sense.

Asking people with good abs about the secret of their success is similar to asking a person with a nice smile about dental care. Even if they are honest, they often attribute it to the wrong reasons.

There can be a number of explanations. An obvious one is your aerobic instructor picked the right parents. Another possible source of the lady's superior definition is some high tension activity she engages in, rock climbing or weight training, for instance.

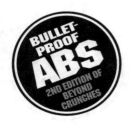

Former Mr. Universe Mike Mentzer had awesome abs in his hey day, yet rarely trained them. His exceptional midriff was the result of heavy squats and dead-lifts. Mentzer worked up to over 1,100 pounds in the quarter squat, and it is obvious that it took a tremendous amount of tension in the muscles of the core to stabilize his spine under such a load.

Q: My calves get sore and sometimes cramp when I work out on the Ab Pavelizer™. What can I do about it?

Strengthen your calves, drink plenty of water and make sure you get enough potassium in your diet. If they still cramp, you may have a health condition.

Q: In my taekwondo class the instructor has us drop medicine balls on each other's stomachs to condition us against kicks and punches. Is this kind of training safe? Is it effective?

No training method is 100% safe. If you do not flex your abs in time, you could conceivably damage your inner organs. It is no different from taking a punch. By the way, in the Soviet Special Forces boot camp drill instructors would hit us in the stomach and expect us to keep a straight face! As I learned later, when it was my turn to punch, it was done mostly for the DIs' amusement. Still, the troopers got desensitized against pain and developed the reflex of bracing up before the impact. While my lawyer would not let me pedal that kind of abuse, I will admit that medicine ball training offers similar benefits in a more controlled environment.

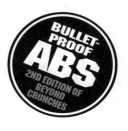

Q: My neck bothers me when I do my ab exercises.
Do you think I should buy an AbRoller?

No.

According to William Kraemer, Ph.D., the president of the National Strength and Conditioning Association, neck support provided by ab training machines creates an unhealthy strength imbalance between the abdominals and the neck muscles. So the neck support is not an asset, but a liability. You haul your head around all day, get used to it!

Anyway, your neck is not likely to tire if you follow the low rep method described in this book.

Q: I feel that most abdominal exercises work my upper abs only.
What about my lower abs?

Please pick up any anatomy book. You will not find either 'lower abs' or 'upper abs'. There is only one long muscle, *rectus abdominis,* connecting your sternum and your pubic bone.

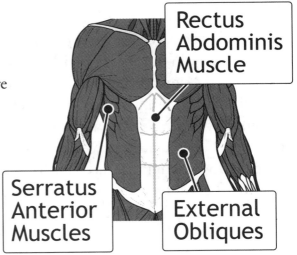

It is impossible to selectively develop a part of a single muscle because of the peculiar way your muscles are hooked up to your brain. Each motor nerve controls its own group of muscle fibers called a motor unit. The constituent fibers are evenly spread out throughout the muscle, rather than being concentrated in its 'peak', or 'sweep', 'lower', or 'upper' part. Even if you manage to recruit a different motor unit with a different exercise, its fibers will still be all over the muscle. So no matter where you attach the load, to your torso, or your legs, you will train the entire length of the abdominal muscle.

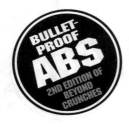

The different sensations that you experience in a muscle from training it at various angles are either from localized constriction of the blood vessels, or mechanical stretching of the tissues on the loaded end of the muscle. Neither is relevant to improving your muscle tone.

Q: Will I get results if the only thing I do for my stomach is the Ab Pavelizer™?

Yes. Just make sure to vary the loading parameters every month: sets, reps, weight, rest intervals, and lifting tempo. You could also follow the cycling format from *Power to the People!: Russian Strength Training Secrets for Every American*

Q: Why do you recommend relaxing between reps and even half-reps on many exercises?

Two reasons. First, recall that we focus on muscular tension, not fatigue, to harden the midsection. Taking a short break between the reps enables you to delay the onset of fatigue and to better focus on tension. Second, relaxing your muscles between bouts of high tension helps to normalize your blood pressure (which does not let you off the medical check-up hook if you are hypertensive or have heart problems). Of course, some exercises, e.g. the Saxon Side Bend, do not provide you with the luxury of taking a break in the middle of a rep.

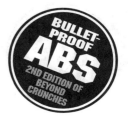

Q: I heard that the abs do not work beyond thirty degrees off the floor. Why do you insist on having people sit up all the way when doing various situps?

The angle you mention is the point at which the spine stops flexing and the abs stop performing dynamic work. They still exert static tension to stabilize the spine and work against the resistance of the viscera if you employ power breathing. Because stabilization is their primary function—unless you are a logger—it is logical to train them consistent with that function. Besides, you earn a breather, which helps your cause.

Q: Is it true that the key to cut up abs is low body fat?

Although high body fat prevents you from displaying your abs to their best advantage, leanness alone will not give you that shredded look. Just check out the abs of a marathon runner to finish that argument once and for all.

Q: Why don't you give any advice on diet and aerobic exercise?

I prefer sticking to the subjects I know. Weight loss is not one of them. Still, I cannot help giving my five roubles. Cut the starches and sugars out of your diet and bump up the protein intake beyond the pencil-neck geek recommendations! No, I am not a Dr. Atkins' fan, I just read classical Russian literature (or at least my lovely wife Julie does).

"Vronsky came to the regimental mess for his beefsteak earlier than usual," wrote Leo Tolstoy in *Anna Karenina* over a century ago. "There was no need for him to follow strict training, since his weight came in just under the regulation hundred-sixty pounds; but he had to avoid getting fat too, and he avoided sweet and starchy food."

Words to live by.

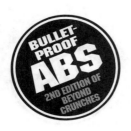

Laying off the carbs and digging your teeth into some steak will also make you a happier and more adjusted person. If you consumed the high carb/low protein chow at a Soviet Special Forces boot camp or in a Lubyanka KGB basement, you would have had an easier time relating to this sentiment.

The carbohydrate-based/protein-restricted diet was scientifically designed to mess with your seratonin and other neurotransmitters. It was an integral part of a brain washing master plan. Its other devious measures included a severe disturbance of your habitual schedule and lifestyle; extreme sleep deprivation; never-ending lies, betrayals, and unpleasant surprises; threats, humiliation, and violence. In addition to this 'standard military package' KGB prisoners also received neuroleptics and other will-suppressing and consciousness-altering drugs.

Your rice cakes and Cheerios are in real friendly company, aren't they?

Q: *When will I see results?*

Immediately. Friedrich Nietzsche said, "The abdomen is the reason a man does not easily mistake himself for a god." Not any more. In a couple of months of *Bullet-Proof Abs* training you may be mistaken for a Greek god or goddess!

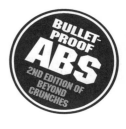

About the Author

Pavel

Pavel Tsatsouline, Master of Sports, was voted *Rolling Stone's* 'Hot Trainer' of the year in 2001. 'The Evil Russian' is the author of a number of best selling fitness books including *Super Joints* and *Power to the People!* He is a contributing editor for Muscle Media magazine.

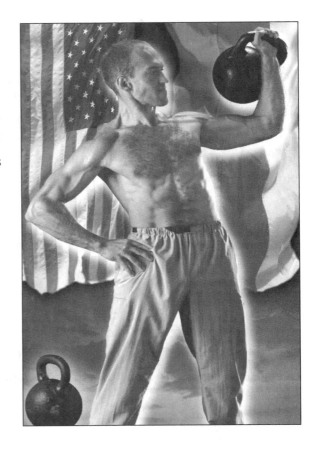

A former Soviet Special Forces instructor, Pavel was nationally ranked in the Russian ethnic sport of kettlebell lifting and holds a Soviet Physical Culture Institute degree in physiology and coaching. Tsatsouline teaches his *'low tech/high concept'* fitness approach to US military and law enforcement agencies and conducts national kettlebell instructor certification courses. Pavel has been interviewed by CNN Headline News, the Fox News Channel, USA Today, Associated Press, and EXTRA TV.

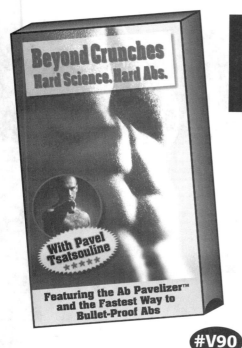

Beyond Crunches
Hard Science. Hard Abs.

With Pavel Tsatsouline
★★★★★

Featuring the Ab Pavelizer™ and the Fastest Way to Bullet-Proof Abs

#V90

BEYOND CRUNCHES

By Pavel Tsatsouline
Video, Running time: 37 min

$29.95   **#V90**

"An Iron Curtain Has Descended Across Your Abs"

Possess a maximum impact training tool for the world's most effective abs, no question. Includes detailed follow-along instructions on how to perform most of the exercises described in the companion book, *Bullet-Proof Abs* Demonstrates advanced techniques for optimizing results with the Ab Pavelizer.

As a former Soviet Union Special Forces conditioning coach, **Pavel Tsatsouline** already knew a thing or two about how to create bullet-stopping abs. Since then, he has combed the world to pry out this select group of primevally powerful ab exercises—guaranteed to yield the fastest, most effective results known to man.

- Fry your abs without the spine-wrecking, neck-jerking stress of traditional crunches.
- No one—but no one—has ever matched Bruce Lee's ripped-beyond-belief abs. What was his favorite exercise? Here it is. Now you can rip your own abs to eye-popping shreds and reclassify yourself as superhuman.
- Russian fighters used this drill, *The Full-Contact Twist,* to increase their striking power and toughen their midsections against blows. An awesome exercise for iron-clad obliques.
- Rapidly download extreme intensity into your situps—with explosive breathing secrets from Asian martial arts.
- Employ a little-known secret from East German research to radically strengthen your situp.
- Do the right thing with "the evil wheel", hit the afterburners and rocket from half-baked to fully-fried abs.
- "Mercy Me!" your obliques will scream when you torture them with the *Saxon Side Bend.*
- How and why to <u>never, never</u> be nice to your abs—and why they'll love you for it.
- A complete workout plan for optimizing your results from the Janda situp and other techniques.

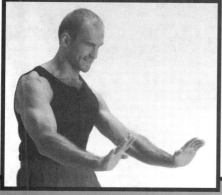

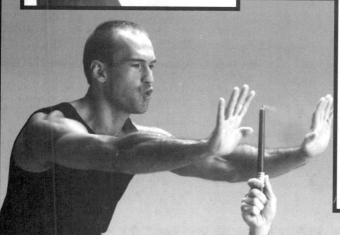

(Right) Pavel's Ab-strengthening breath techniques will give you the power to explode a water bottle—but don't try this trick at home—if the extreme air-pressure whacks back into your lungs, instead of exploding the water bottle—you can end up very dead, which is a bummer for everyone.

(Left) Pavel demonstrates the Power Breathing technique *Bending the Fire* to develop an extra edge in your abs training.

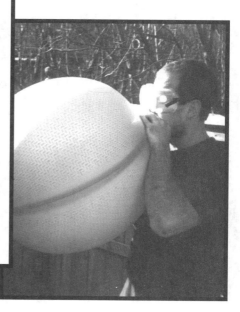

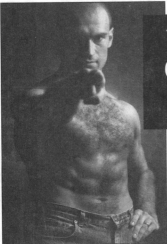

"New Ab Machine Exposes Frauds, Fakes and Cheaters–But Rewards Faithful with the Most Spectacular Abs This Side of Heaven"

The Ab Pavelizer™ II
Item # P12

$130.00
**10-25 lb Olympic plate required for correct use.
(You will need to supply your own plate)**

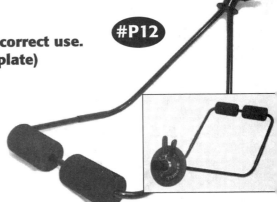

#P12

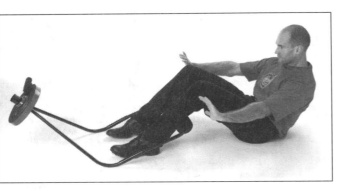

You know, it's a crying shame to cheat on your abs. Your abs are your very core, your center. Your abs define you, man or woman. So why betray them with neglect and less-than-honest carryings-on? That's bad! And everybody always knows! Rationalize all you want, hide all you want, but weak, flabby abs scream your lack of self-respect to all comers. Why live at all, if you can't hold your head up high and own a flat stomach?

Fortunately, you can now come clean, get honest and give your abs the most challenging, yet rewarding workout of their lives. And believe me, they will love you for ever!

Maybe you've been misled. Maybe you think you have to flog out hundreds of situps to get spectacular abs? Ho! Sorry, **but with abs, repetition is the mother of insanity.** Forget about it! You're just wasting your time! You're just fooling around! No wonder you're still not satisfied!

No, if you <u>really, really</u> want abs-to-die-for then: INTENSITY IS EVERYTHING!

FREE BONUS:

Comes with a four page detailed instruction guide on how to use and get the most out of your Ab Pavelizer™ II. Includes two incredible methods for massively intensifying your ab workout with *Power* and *Paradox Breathing*.

And here lies the secret of **The Ab Pavelizer™ II.** It's all in the extreme, unavoidable intensity it thrusts on you. No room for skulkers or shirkers. No room at all! Either get with the program or slink back under the stone from under which you crept.

You see, The Ab Pavelizer™ II's new sleek-'n-light design guarantees a perfect sit-up by forcing you to do it right. Now, escape or half-measures are impossible. Sit down at the Ab Pavelizer™ II and a divine slab of abs will be served up whether you like it or not. You'll startle yourself in your own mirror!

The secret to the Ab Pavelizer™ II is in the **extra-active** resistance it provides you. The cunning device literally pushes up against your calves (you'd almost swear it was a cruel, human partner) and forces you to recruit your glutes and hamstrings.

Two wonderful and amazing things happen.

First, it is virtually impossible to do the Janda situp wrong unless you start with a jerk. Second, the exercise becomes MUCH harder than on the Ab Pavelizer™ Classic. And "Much Harder" is Russian for "Quicker Results."

It is astonishingly hard to sit up all the way when the new Ab Pavelizer™ II is loaded with enough weight, 10-35 pounds for most comrades. If you can do three sets of five reps you will already have awesome abs.

A Great Added Benefit: Are you living in an already over-cluttered space? Want to conveniently hide the secret of your abs-success from envious neighbors? The new Ab Pavelizer™ II easily and quickly folds away in a closet or under your bed. Once prying eyes have left, you can put it up again in seconds for another handshake with heaven—or hell, depending on your perspective.

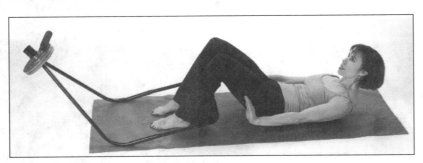

1•800•899•5111 24 HOURS A DAY, OR FAX: (866) 280-7619

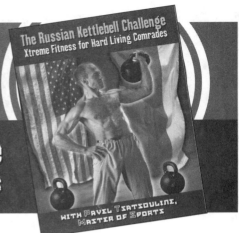
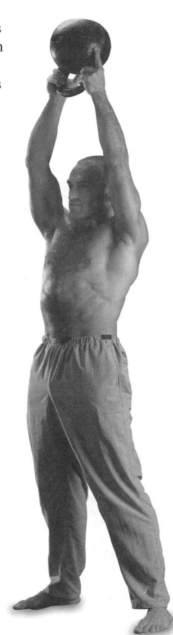
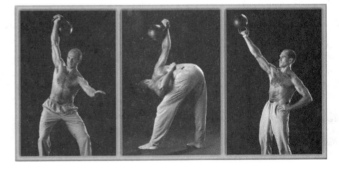

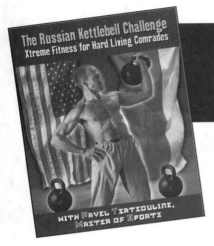

Section One
The History of the Russian Kettlebell—How and Why a Low-Tech Ball of Iron Became the National Choice for Super-Tech Results

Vodka, pickle juice, kettlebell lifting, and other Russian pastimes

'The working class sport'

Finally: Xtreme all around fitness!
Why Soviet science considers kettlebells to be one of the best tools for all around physical development....

Kettlebells in the Red Army
The Red Army catches on.... every Russian military unit equipped with K-bells....the perfect physical conditioning for military personnel....the vital combination of strength and endurance....*Girevoy sport* delivers unparalleled cardio benefits....why *Spetznaz* personnel owe much of their wiry strength, explosive agility, and stamina to kettlebells....

Section Two
Special Applications—How The Russian Kettlebell Can Dramatically Enhance Your Chosen Endeavor

Kettlebells for combat sports
Russian wrestlers do lion's share of conditioning with kettlebells.... Why KB one arm snatches work better than Hindu squats....KB's strengthen respiratory muscles.... boxers appreciate newfound ability to keep on punching....KB's reduce shoulder injuries.... develop the ability to absorb ballistic shocks....build serious tendons and ligaments in wrists, elbows, shoulders, and back—with power to match....why kettlebell drills are better than plyometrics as a tool for developing power....KB's the tool of choice for rough sports.

Why Russian lifters train with kettlebells
Famous Soviet weightlifters start Olympic careers with KB's.... Olympic weightlifters add KB's for spectacular gains in shoulder and hip flexibility.... for developing quickness.... overhead kettlebell squats unmatchable in promoting hip and lower back flexibility for powerlifters....

Get huge with kettlebells—if you wish
Why the *girya* is superior to the dumbbell or barbell, for arm and chest training....how to gain muscle size doing KB J&J's.... repetition one arm snatches for bulking up your back, shoulders, and biceps.... incorporating KB's into drop sets—for greater mass and vascularity.

Kettlebells for arm-wrestlers
World champion arm wrestler gives KB's two thumbs up....why the kettlebell is one of the best grip and forearm developers in existence....

Getting younger and healthier with kettlebells
The amazing health benefits of KB training....Doctor Krayevskiy's 20-year age-reversal....successful rehabilitation of hopeless back injuries with kettlebells.... Valentin Dikul—from broken back to All Time Historic Deadlift of 460kg, thanks to KB's.... why KB's can be highly beneficial for your joints.

How kettlebells melt fat and build a powerful heart—without the dishonor of dieting and aerobics
Spectacular fat loss....enhanced metabolism....increased growth hormone....a remarkable decrease in heart rates....

Section Three
Doing It—Kettlebell Techniques and Programs for Xtreme Fitness

Why Kettlebells?
The many reasons to choose K-bells over mainstream equipment and methods.... KBs suitable for men and women young and old.... perfect for military, law enforcement and athletic teams.... *Giryas*—a 'working class' answer to weightlifting and plyometrics promoting shoulder and hip flexibility....best bet for building best-at-show muscles.... highly effective for strengthening the connective tissues....fixing bad backs....cheap and virtually indestructible....promotes genuine 'all-around fitness' —strength, explosiveness, flexibility, endurance, and fat loss.

The program minimum

The Russian Kettlebell Challenge workout: the program-maximum
Pavel's own free style program....the top ten Russian Kettlebell Challenge training guidelines....how often and how long to train.... The secret key to successful frequent training.... THE most effective tool of strength development....difficulty and intensity variation.... how to add *Power to the People!* and other drills to your kettlebell regimen

The kettlebell drills: *Explode!*
- **Swing/snatch pull**
- **Clean**—The key to efficient and painless shock absorption.... making the clean tougher....the pure evil of the two K-bells clean.... seated hang cleans, for gorilla traps and shoulders....
- **Snatch**—The one-arm snatch—Tsar of kettlebell lifts
- **Under the leg pass**—A favorite of the Russian military—great for the midsection
- **Jerk, Clean & Jerk**
- **Jump shrug**

The kettlebell drills: *Grind!*
- **Military press**—How to add and maximize tension for greater power....One hundred wa to cook the military press ... The negative press....the 'powerlifter's secret weapon for maxima results in your lifts....why to lift what you can't lift.... the graduated press....how to get more out of a 'light' weight.... the two-kettlebells press.... technique for building strength and musc mass....the 'waiter press' for strict and perfect pressing skill....
- **Floor pullover and press**
- **Good morning stretch**—Favored by Russian weightlifters, for spectacular hamstring flexibility and hip strength.
- **Windmill**—An unreal drill for a powerful and flexible waist, back, and hips.
- **Side press**—A potent mix of the windmill and the military press—"one of the best builders of the shoulders and upper back."
- **Bent press**—A favorite lift of Eugene Sandow's—and The Evil One.... why the bes built men in history have been bent pressers....leads to proficiency in all other lifts....how to simultaneously use every muscle in your body.... A Brazilian Jiu Jitsu champion's personal kettlebell program

Section Four
Classic Kettlebell Programs from Mother Russia
The official Soviet weightlifting textbook *girevoy sport* system of training

The *Weightlifting Yearbook girevoy sport* programs

Three official armed forces *girevoy sport* programs

Group training with kettlebells—Red Army style

Xtreme kettlebell training—Russian Navy SEAL style
Performing snatches and other explosive kettlebell drills under water....pseudo-isokinetic resistance.... how to make your muscle fibers blast into action faster than ever....

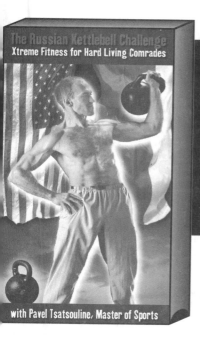

#V103

with Pavel Tsatsouline, Master of Sports

The Russian Kettlebell Challenge

Xtreme Fitness for Hard Living Comrades

with Pavel Tsatsouline, Master of Sports

Item # V103 $39.95
Video Running Time: 32 minutes

If you are looking for a supreme edge in your chosen sport—seek no more!

Both the Soviet Special Forces and numerous world-champion Soviet Olympic athletes used the ancient Russian Kettlebell as their secret weapon for xtreme fitness. Thanks to the kettlebells's astonishing ability to turbocharge physical performance, these Soviet supermen creamed their opponents time-and-time-again, with inhuman displays of raw power and explosive strength.

Now, former Spetznaz trainer, international fitness author and nationally ranked kettlebell lifter, Pavel Tsatsouline, delivers this secret Soviet weapon into your own hands.

You <u>NEVER have to be second best again!</u> Here is the first-ever complete kettlebell training program—for Western shock-attack athletes who refuse to be denied—and who'd rather be dead than number two.

- **Get really, really nasty—with a commando's wiry strength, the explosive agility of a tiger and the stamina of a world-class iron-man.**

- **Own the single best conditioning tool for killer sports like kick-boxing, wrestling, and football.**

- **Watch in amazement as high-rep kettle-bells let you hack the fat off your meat—without the dishonor of aerobics and dieting**

- **Kick your fighting system into warp speed—with high-rep snatches and clean-and-jerks**

- **Develop steel tendons and ligaments—and a whiplash power to match**

- **Effortlessly absorb ballistic shocks—and laugh as you shrug off the hardest hits your opponent can muster**

- **Go ape on your enemies—with gorilla shoulders and tree-swinging traps**

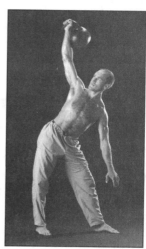

An ancient Russian exercise device, the kettlebell has long been a favorite in that country for those seeking a special edge in strength and endurance.

It was the key in forging the mighty power of dinosaurs like Ivan "the Champion of Champions", Poddubny. Poddubny, one of the strongest men of his time, trained with kettlebells in preparation for his undefeated wrestling career and six world champion belts.

Many famous Soviet weightlifters, such as Vorobyev, Vlasov, Alexeyev, and Stogov, started their Olympic careers with old-fashioned kettlebells.

Kettlebells come in "poods". A pood is an old Russian measure of weight, which equals 16kg, or 36 pounds. There are one, one and a half, and two pood K-bells, 16, 24, and 32kg respectively.

To earn his national ranking, Pavel Tsatsouline had to power snatch a 32kg kettlebell forty times with one arm, and forty with the other back to back and power clean and jerk two such bells forty-five times.

Soviet science discovered that repetition kettlebell lifting is one of the best tools for all around physical development. (Voropayev, 1983) observed two groups of college students over a period of a few years. A standard battery of the armed forces PT tests was used: pullups, a standing broad jump, a 100m sprint, and a 1k run. The control group followed the typical university physical training program which was military oriented and emphasized the above exercises. The experimental group just lifted kettlebells. In spite of the lack of practice on the tested drills, the KB group showed better scores in every one of them.

The Red Army, too pragmatic to waste their troopers, time on pushups and situps, quickly caught on. Every Russian military unit's gym was equipped with K-bells. Spetznaz, Soviet Special Operations, personnel owe much of their wiry strength, explosive agility, and never quitting stamina to kettlebells. High rep C&Js and snatches with K-bells kick the fighting man,s system into warp drive.

In addition to their many mentioned benefits, the official kettlebell lifts also develop the ability to absorb ballistic shocks. If you want to develop your ability to take impact try the official K-bell lifts. The repetitive ballistic shock builds extremely strong tendons and ligaments.

The ballistic blasts of kettlebell lifting become an excellent conditioning tool for athletes from rough sports like kick-boxing, wrestling, and football. And the extreme metabolic cost of high rep KB workouts will put your unwanted fat on a fire sale.

Look WAY YOUNGER than Your Age
Have a LEAN, GRACEFUL, Athletic-Looking Body
Feel AMAZING, Feel VIGOROUS, Feel BEAUTIFUL
Have MORE Energy and MORE Strength to
Get MORE Done in Your Day

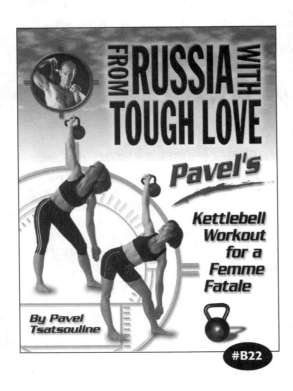

From Russia with Tough Love
Pavel's Kettlebell Workout for a Femme Fatale
Book By Pavel Tsatsouline

Paperback 184 pages 8.5" x 11"

#B22 $34.95

In Russia, kettlebells have long been revered as the fitness-tool of choice for Olympic athletes, elite special forces and martial artists. The kettlebell's ballistic movement challenges the body to achieve an unparalleled level of physical conditioning and overall strength.

But until now, the astonishing benefits of the Russian kettlebell have been unavailable to all but a few women. Kettlebells have mostly been the sacred preserve of the male professional athlete, the military and other hardcore types. That's about to change, as Russian fitness expert and best selling author PAVEL, delivers the first-ever kettlebell program for women.

It's wild, but women really CAN have it all when they access the magical power of Russian kettlebells. Pavel's uncompromising workouts give *across-the-board, simultaneous, spectacular and immediate results* for all aspects of physical fitness: strength, speed, endurance, fat-burning, you name it. Kettlebells deliver any and everything a woman could want—if she wants to be in the best-shape-ever of her life.

And one handy, super-simple tool—finally available in woman-friendly sizes—does it all. No bulky, expensive machines. No complicated gizmos. No time-devouring trips to the gym.

Into sports? Jump higher. Leap further. Kick faster. Hit harder. Throw harder. Run with newfound speed. Swim with greater power. Endure longer. Wow!

Working hard? Handle stress with ridiculous ease. Blaze thru tasks in half the time. Radiate confidence. Knock 'em dead with your energy and enthusiasm.

Can't keep up with your kids? Not any more! They won't know what hit them.

Just wanna have fun? Feel super-relaxed from the endorphin-rush of your life, dance all night and feel finer-than-fine the next morning...and the next...and the next.

Got attitude? Huh! Then try Pavel's patented Russian Kettlebell workouts. Now, THAT'S attitude!

Just some of what From Russia with Tough Love reveals:

- How the *Snatch* eliminates cellulite, firms your butt, and gives you the cardio-ride of a lifetime
- How to get as strong as you want, without bulking up
- How the *Swing* melts your fat and blasts your hips 'n thighs
- How to supercharge your heart and lungs without aerobics
- How to shrink your waist with the *Power Breathing Crunch*
- How the *Deck Squat* makes you super flexible
- An incredible exercise to tone your arms and shoulders
- The *Clean-and-Press*—for a magnificent upper body
- *The real secret to great muscle tone*
- The *Overhead Squat* for explosive leg strength
- How to *think* yourself stronger—yes, really!
- The queen of situps—for those who can hack it
- Cool combination exercises that deliver an unbelievable muscular and cardiovascular workout in zero time
- An unreal drill for a powerful and flexible waist, back, and hips
- How to perform multiple mini-sessions for fast-lane fitness

"Download this tape into your eager cells and watch in stunned disbelief as your body reconstitutes itself, almost overnight"

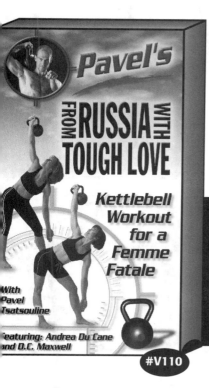

#V110

From Russia with Tough Love

Pavel's Kettlebell Workout
for a Femme Fatale
With Pavel Tsatsouline
VIDEO Running Time: 1hr 12 minutes
#V110 $29.95

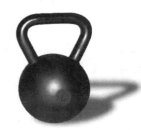

The Sure-Fire Secret to Looking Younger, Leaner and Stronger AND Having More Energy to Get a Whole Lot More Done in the Day

What you'll discover when "Tough" explodes on your monitor:

- The *Snatch*—to eliminate cellulite, firm your butt, and give you the cardio-workout of a lifetime
- The *Swing*— to fry your fat and slenderize hips 'n thighs
- The *Power Breathing Crunch*—to shrink your waist
- The *Deck Squat*—for strength and super-flexiblity
- An incredible exercise to tone your arms and shoulders
- The *Clean-and-Press*—for a magnificent upper body
- The *Overhead Squat*—for explosive leg strength
- The queen of situps—for a flat, flat stomach
- Combination exercises that wallop you with an unbelievable muscular and cardio workout

Spanking graphics, a kick-ass opening, smooth-as-silk camera work, Pavel at his absolute dynamic best, two awesome femme fatales, and a slew of fantastic KB exercises, many of which were not included on the original Russian Kettlebell Challenge video.

At one hour and twenty minutes of rock-solid, cutting-edge information, this video is value-beyond-belief. I challenge any woman worth her salt not to be able to completely transform herself physically with this one tape.

"In six weeks of kettlebell work, I lost an inch off my waist and dropped my heart rate 6 beats per minute, while staying the same weight. I was already working out when I started using kettlebells, so I'm not a novice. There are few ways to lose fat, gain muscle, and improve your cardio fitness all at the same time; I've never seen a better one than this."
—*Steven Justus, Westminster, CO*

"Kettlebells are without a doubt the most effective strength/endurance conditioning tool out there. I wish I had known about them 15 years ago!"
—*Santiago, Orlando, FL*

"I have practiced Kettlebell training for a year and a half. I now have an anatomy chart back and have gotten MUCH stronger."
—*Samantha Mendelson, Coral Gables, FL*

"I know now that I will never walk into a gym again - who would? It is absolutely amazing how much individual accomplishment can be attained using a kettlebell. Simply fantastic. I would recommend it to anyone at any fitness level, in any sport.
—*William Hevener, North Cape May, NJ*

"It is the most effective training tool I have ever used. I have increased both my speed and endurance, with extra power to boot. It wasn't even a priority, but I lost some bodyfat, which was nice. However, increased athletic performance was my main goal, and this is where the program really shines."
—*Tyler Hass, Walla Walla, WA*

Russian Kettlebells—The Ultimate Iron Game for Massive, Massive, Massive, Massive, Massive
RESULTS

"I've been working out with weights for over 25 years, and **The Russian Kettlebell Challenge** is simply the best approach I've ever found to combining strength training, endurance, and flexibility. Pavel Tsatsouline has done his usual outstanding job of presenting clear, no-nonsense info on the best way to get into killer shape, with tremendous carryover for virtually any athletic endeavor. The companion video for this book is superb as well, and a must for mastering some of the nuances of the unique kettlebell exercises. I have purchased almost all of Pavel's excellent works, and they have literally changed my life. Now, I'm addicted to kettlebell training, and more excited and enthusiastic about working out than ever. **The Russian Kettlebell Challenge** is Pavel's best work yet - and that's saying a lot. I highly recommend this book, and all of Pavel's products. If you're serious about exercise and getting into the best shape of your life with surprising ease, you will not be disappointed with this or any of Pavel's products."—John Quigley, Hazleton, PA

"**The Russian Kettlebell Challenge** companion book and video are well-crafted and user-friendly re-introductions to the lost (in America) art of kettle-bell lifting. I am in my late 40's and have been physically active all my adult life in a range of activities, including running and cardio kickboxing when they were trendy, as well as biking, swimming, running, weightlifting, various ball sports, etc. None of those activities has been as much fun, or as productive, as RKC. I highly recommend Pavel's RKC book and video, and kettlebell lifting in general."
—**Gary Karl, Rochester, NY**

"Wow, I have always been a fan of Pavel's books. However, this is his best book yet! I have been doing Kettlebell training for two months and love it. It is one of the best methods to acquire functional strength and is really enjoyable. I can see clearly how it would be beneficial to martial artists and strength athletes such as powerlifters and especially Olympic weightlifters."—**Mike Mahler, McLean, VA**

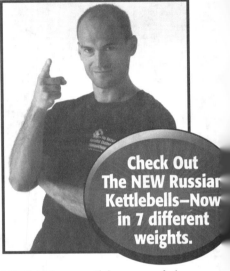

Check Out The NEW Russsiar Kettlebells—Now in 7 different weights.

"This is possibly one of the best fitness books I have ever read! I train strictly with Kettlebells and it's taken me to inhuman levels of fitness and strength. Throw off the shackles of easy living and become a living, breathing chunk of steel!"—**Daniel J. Rodgers, Moscow, ID**

"As a karateka, I have found that kettlebell training has improved my hand speed, foot speed, and striking power, and has made me tougher to hit and tougher to hurt. To my knowledge no other type of training will do that all at once."— **Robert Lawrence, Brooklyn, NY**

1•800•899•5111   24 HOURS A DAY, OR FAX: (866) 280-7619

AMAZING NEWS:
ow You Can Carry a Whole Gym
One Hand—and Get a Fabulous,
OTAL WORKOUT
ght in Your Own Living Room

picture-perfect slen-

lean, lean
cle tone

way-faster fat loss

firmer hips,
hs and butt

into the
mest, coolest, slinki-
clothes

looked at twice—and
some

the bust line you
rve and want

a tremendous aerobic
kout in half the time
used to take

Each Russian Kettlebell is manufactured exclusively by Dragon Door Publications. The new kettlebells have a steel handle and a steel core surrounded by a rubber ball. These kettlebells are designed to last a lifetime—and beyond.

Special warning: Treat your kettlebell lifting with the utmost care, precision and respect. Watch Pavel's kettle-bell video many, many times for perfect form and correct execution. If possible, sign up for one of Pavel's upcoming

Russian Kettlebell Challenge workshops.

Lift at your own discretion! We are not responsible for you boinking yourself on the head, dropping it on your feet or any other politically-incorrect action. Stick to the Party line, Comrade!

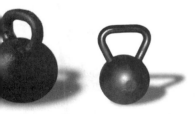
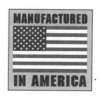

MANUFACTURED IN AMERICA

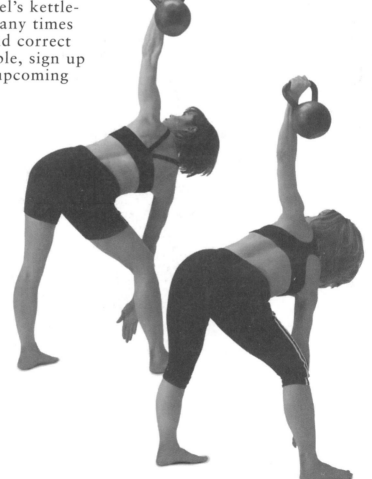

SIAN KETTLEBELLS

ESIGNED FOR WOMEN

4kg (approx. 9 lb)	$89.95	S/H: $10.00
8kg (approx. 18 lb)	$99.95	S/H: $14.00

ther notice, these new kettlebells are not available

C KETTLEBELLS

12kg (approx. 26lb)	$82.95	S/H: $20.00
16kg (approx. 35lb)	$89.95	S/H: $24.00
24kg (approx. 53lb)	$109.95	S/H: $32.00
32kg (approx. 70lb)	$139.95	S/H: $39.00

40kg SIZE—HEAVY METAL!

40kg (approx. 88lb)	$179.95	S/H: $52.00

ORDER A SET OF CLASSIC KETTLEBELLS AND
7.00!

Set, one of A, B & C—16, 24 & 32kg.		
(Save $17.00)	$322.85	S/H: $95.00

The Russian Kettlebells are only available to customers resident in the U.S. mainland. Normal shipping charges do not apply. No rush orders on kettlebells.

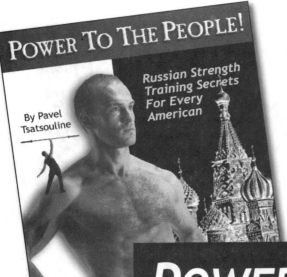

POWER TO THE PEOPLE!

RUSSIAN STRENGTH TRAINING SECRETS FOR EVERY AMERICAN

By Pavel Tsatsouline

8½" x 11" 124 pages, over 100 photographs and illustrations—$34.95 #B10

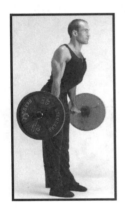

How would you like to own a world class body—<u>whatever your present condition</u>— by doing only two exercises, for twenty minutes a day?" A body so lean, ripped and powerful looking, you won't believe your own reflection when you catch yourself in the mirror.

And what if you could do it without a single supplement, without having to waste your time at a gym and with only a 150 bucks of simple equipment?

And how about not only being stronger than you've ever been in your life, but having higher energy and better performance in whatever you do?

How would you like to have an instant download of the world's <u>absolutely most effective strength secrets?</u> To possess exactly the same knowledge that created world-champion athletes—and the strongest bodies of their generation?"

Pavel Tsatsouline's *Power to the People!— Russian Strength Training Secrets for Every American* delivers all of this and more.

As **Senior Science Editor for Joe Weider's** *Flex* **magazine, Jim Wright** is recognized as one of the world's premier authorities on strength training. Here's more of what he had to say:

Here's just some of what you'll discover, when you possess your own copy of Pavel Tsatsouline's *Power to the People!*:

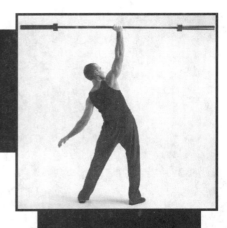

- How to get super strong without training to muscle failure or exhaustion
- How to hack into your 'muscle software' and magnify your power and muscle definition
- How to get super strong <u>without putting on an ounce of weight</u>
- Or how to build massive muscles with a classified Soviet Special Forces workout
- Why high rep training to the 'burn' is like a form of rigor mortis—and what it really takes to develop spectacular muscle tone
- How to mold your whole body into an off-planet rock with only two exercises
- How to increase your bench press by ten pounds overnight
- How to design a world class body in your basement—with $150 worth of basic weights and in twenty minutes a day
- How futuristic techniques can squeeze more horsepower out of your body-engine
- How to maximize muscular tension for traffic-stopping muscular definition
- How to minimize fatigue and get the most out of your strength training
- How to ensure high energy after your workout
- How to get stronger and harder without getting bigger
- Why it's safer to use free weights than machines
- How to achieve massive muscles <u>and</u> awesome strength—if that's what you want
- What, how and when to eat for maximum gains
- How to master the magic of effective exercise variation
- The ultimate formula for strength
- How to gain beyond your wildest dreams—with less chance of injury
- A high intensity, immediate gratification technique for massive strength gains
- The eight most effective breathing habits for lifting weights
- The secret that separates elite athletes from 'also-rans'
- How to become super strong and live to tell about it

"You are not training if you are not training with Pavel!"

—Dr. Fred Clary, National Powerlifting Champion and World Record Holder.

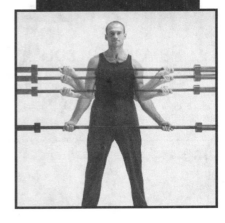

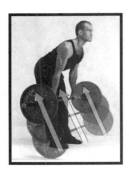

Russians have always made do with simple solutions without compromising the results. NASA aerospace types say that while America sends men to the moon in a Cadillac, Russia manages to launch them into space in a tin can. Enter the tin can approach to designing a world class body—in your basement with $150 worth of equipment. After all, US gyms are stuffed with hi-tech gear, yet it is the Russians with their metal junkyard training facilities who have dominated the Olympics for decades.

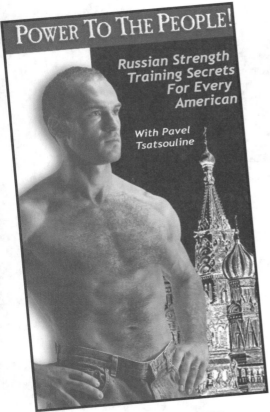

POWER TO THE PEOPLE!

Russian Strength Training Secrets For Every American

With Pavel Tsatsouline

#V102

POWER TO THE PEOPLE

By Pavel Tsatsouline
Video, Running time: 47 min
$29.95   #V102

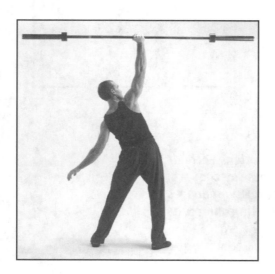

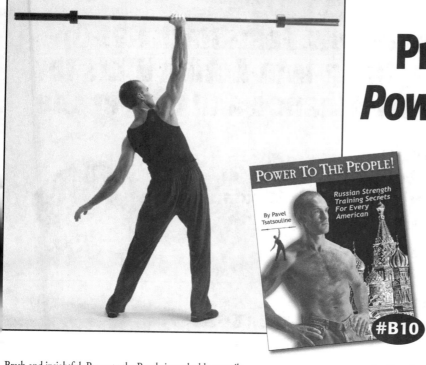

Praise for Pavel's Power to the People!

"In **Power to the People!** Pavel Tsatsouline reveals an authentically Russian approach to physical fitness. He shows how anyone, by learning how to contract their muscles harder, can build up to incredible levels of strength without gaining an ounce of weight. He shows how to exercise with a super-strict form and lift more weight than can be accomplished by swing or cheat. Now it's possible to train the human body to world-class fitness standards at home, working out for twenty minutes a day, and with only $150.00 worth of basic weights. **Power to the People!** is a highly recommended addition to any personal or professional physical fitness reference bookshelf."—**Midwest Book Review, Oregon, WI**

Brash and insightful, Power to the People is a valuable compilation of how-to strength training information. Pavel Tsatsouline offers a fresh and provocative perspective on resistance training, and charts a path to self-improvement that is both practical and elegantly simple. If building strength is your top priority, then *Power to the People* belongs at the top of your reading list. —**Rob Faigin, author of Natural Hormonal Enhancement**

"I learned a lot from Pavel's books and plan to use many of his ideas in my own workouts. *Power to the People!* is an eye-opener. It will give you new—and valuable—perspectives on strength training. You will find plenty of ideas here to make your training more productive."—**Clarence Bass, author of Ripped 1, 2 &3.**

"A good book for the athlete looking for a routine that will increase strength without building muscle mass. Good source of variation for anyone who's tired of doing standard exercises."—**Jonathan Lawson, IronMan Magazine**

"I have been a training athlete for over 30 years. I played NCAA basketball in college, kick boxed as a pro for two years, made it to the NFL as a free agent in 1982, powerlifted through my 20's and do Olympic lifting now at 42. I have also coached swimming and strength athletes for over 20 years.I have never read a book more useful than **Power to the People!** I have seen my strength explode like I was in my 20's again—and my joints are no longer hurting."—**Carter Stamm, New Orleans, LA**

"I have been following a regimen I got from *Power to the People!* for about seven weeks now. I have lost about 17lbs and have lost three inches in my waist. My deadlift has gone from a meager 180lbs to 255 lbs in that short time as well."—**Lawrence J. Kochert**

Like *Beyond Stretching* and *Beyond Crunches*, his other books, this is great. I think that it is the best book on effective strength training that I have ever read. This is not a book just about theory and principles. But Tsatsouline provides a detailed and complete outline of an exact program to do and how to customize it for yourself. It is very different from anything you have probably every read about strength training. The things he teaches in the book though won't just get you strong, if you want more than that, but can make you look really good—lean, ripped, and/or real big muscled if you want it. It's a very good book; the best available English-language print matter on the topic of strength training."—**Dan Paltzik**

The great thing about the book *"Power to the People!"* is that it tells the readers what not to do when training for strength and why not. As you read the book, you will keep saying to yourself: "so that's why I'm not getting stronger!" Pavel points out all the things that are wrong with conventional weight training (and there is lots of it) and shows the readers what they need to do to get stronger, but not necessarily bigger."— **Sang Kim, Rome, GA**

Using Pavel Tsatsouline's weight training methods from his book *Power to the People* gives you the feeling that you can take on the world after only a 20-30 minute workout! Tsatsouline's book is written with such cleverness, clarity, and detail that I couldn't put it down. I am thoroughly enthusiastic about weight training where my past indoor training consisted only of Yoga postures. I would recommend this book to anyone interested in enhancing their performance on the job, in weight training, and in other athletic pursuits.

Pavel's genius is that he can take a complex subject like weight training and design a program that is enjoyable, efficient and gets fast results. He has done the same thing for abdominal development and stretching."—**Cliff D.V., Honolulu, Hawaii**

"I have experienced Pavel Tsatsouline's methods up close and in person, and his scientific approach lays waste to the muscleheaded garbage that we've been conditioned to follow. Pavel will show you how to achieve a full-body workout with just two core exercises and $150 worth of barbell equipment. You won't get injured and you won't get stiff. You'll just get what you were looking for in the first place - a program that works and one that you'll stick with." — **David M Gaynes, Bellevue, WA**

"It isn't growth hormone... it's Pavel! This is THE definitive text on the art and science of strength training... and that's what it's all about, power! Page after page of the world's most useful and productive strength-training practices are explained in this book. A lot of experienced lifters, who think that they know how to train, will be humbled when they find out how much better Pavel's system is than anything the western iron-game community has ever done. I have surpassed all my previous bests...and I no longer need or use lifting belts. I learned how to up-regulate tension through his "feed-forward" technique, how to immediately add AT LEAST ten pounds to every lift via "hyperirradiation", and to do it in my best form ever, and how to gain on every lift WEEKLY through the Russian system of periodization without any plateaus! Seriously, I gain every week! You only need TWO exercises! Pavel explains which ones, how to do them and how often. Also, you'll learn how to train to SUCCESS, not to "failure", how to immediately turn any lift into a "hyper lift", teach your nervous system how not to ever "miss" a lift, and simultaneously make your body far less injury-prone! Pavel illustrates the two types of muscle growth and which one you REALLY need, and the all-important power breathing. Pavel's training is the most valuable resource made available for strength athletes since the barbell. The breathing techniques alone are worth the asking price. This book is my personal favorite out of all his works, and in my opinion, they should be owned as a set. This book is superior to all the muscle mags and books that dwell on a content of unessential details of today's "fitness culture" and yet never fully explain the context of training for strength. Pavel cuts right to the heart of the "muscle mystery", by explaining the all-important context of the Russian system: quick, efficient, permanent strength gains, without spending a small fortune on "me-too" bodybuilding supplements and without unnecessary, time consuming overtraining. Now I only hope he writes a book on full-contact training..."—**Sean Williams, Long Beach, NY**

"This is a real source of no-b.s. information on how to build strength without adding bulk. I learned some new things which one can't find in books like *'Beyond Brawn'* or *'Dinosaur Training'*. Perhaps an advanced powerlifter, who reads Milo, already knows all that stuff, but I would definitely recommend this book to everyone from beginners to intermediates who are interested in increasing their strength."
—**Nikolai Pastouchenko, Tallahassee, Florid**

"Forget all of the fancy rhetoric. If you are serious about improving your strength and your health buy this book and pay attention to what's provided. I started in January 2000 doing deadlifts with 200 lbs. Three months later I was at 365 lbs. Pavel knows what he is talking about and knows how to explain it simply. That's it."—**Alan, Indiana**

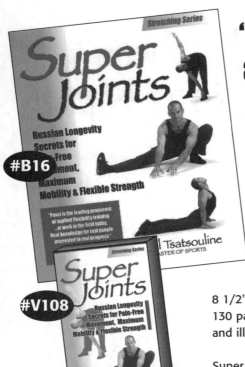

"The Do-It-Now, Fast-Start, Get-Up-and-Go, Jump-into-Action Bible for High Performance and Longer Life"

Super Joints
Russian Longevity Secrets for Pain-Free Movement, Maximum Mobility & Flexible Strength

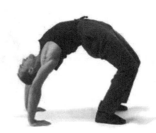

Super Joints Book
by Pavel Tsatsouline
#B16   **$34.95**
8 1/2" x 11" Paperback
130 pages - Over 100 photos
and illustrations

Super Joints Video
with Pavel Tsatsouline
#V108   **$24.95**
Running Time: 33 minutes

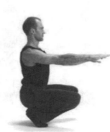

You have a choice in life. You can sputter and stumble and creak your way along in a process of painful, slow decline—or you can take charge of your health and become a human dynamo.

And there is no better way to insure a long, pain-free life than performing the right daily combination of joint mobility and strength-flexibility exercises.

In *Super Joints*, Russian fitness expert Pavel Tsatsouline shows you exactly how to quickly achieve and maintain peak joint health—and then use it to improve every aspect of your physical performance.

Only the foolish would deliberately ignore the life-saving and life-enhancing advice Pavel offers in *Super Joints*. Why would anyone willingly subject themselves to a life of increasing pain, degeneration and decrepitude? But for an athlete, a dancer, a martial artist or any serious performer, *Super Joints* could spell the difference between greatness and mediocrity.

Discover:

- The twenty-eight most valuable drills for youthful joints and a stronger stretch
- How to save your joints and prevent or reduce arthritis
- The one-stop care-shop for your inner Tin Man— how to give your nervous system a tune up, your joints a lube-job and your energy a recharge
- What it takes to go from cruise control to full throttle: The One Thousand Moves Morning Recharge—Amosov's "bigger bang" calisthenics complex for achieving heaven-on earth in 25 minutes
- How to make your body feel better than you can remember—active flexibility fosporting prowess and fewer injuries
- The amazing Pink Panther technique that may add a couple of feet to your stretch the first time you do it

1•800•899•5111
24 HOURS A DAY
FAX YOUR ORDER (866) 280-7619

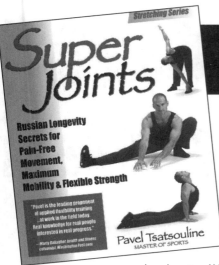

Here's what you'll discover, when you possess your own copy of Pavel Tsatsouline's *Super Joints*

Who needs *Super Joints?*...the needs-based survey for super-healthy joint owners... decreasing the odds of injuries...how to develop the right blend of strength and flexibility and improve your survival odds... for better performance...*active flexibility* versus *passive flexibility*... restoring youthful mobility...flexibility development for young athletes... improving posture...kicking-range...improving passive flexibility.

How to keep your one hundred joints running smooth...how *Mobility Drills* can save your joints and prevent or reduce arthritis ...the *theory of limit loads*...Amosov's daily complex of joint mobility exercises...Lying Behind-the-Head Leg Raises...Standing Toe-Touch...Arm Circles... Side bends...Shoulder Blade Reach...Torso Turn...Knee Raises...Pushups...Roman Chair Situps...how to make the Roman chair situp safer...*paradoxical breathing*...squats... the secrets of safer back bending...Amosov's vital tip for creating a surge in your fountain-of-youth calisthenics.

The distinct difference between *joint mobility* and *muscle flexibility* training...Amosov's "three stages of joint health"...appropriate maintenance/prevention strategies for the three stages...how to get started and how to ramp up....the correct tempos for best results—Amosov's way and Pavel's way...when best to perform your mobility drills... shakin' up your proprioceptors—the one-stop care-shop for your inner Tin Man...how to give your nervous system a tune up, your joints a lube-job and your energy a recharge.

From cruise control to full throttle: *The One Thousand Moves Morning Recharge*—Academician Amosov's "bigger bang" calisthenics complex—how to add more cardio and more strengthening to you joint mobility program...adding One Legged Jumps, Stomach Sucks and *The Birch Tree*—how to achieve heaven-on-earth in 25–40 minutes.

Checking yourself...are your joints mobile enough?—F. L. Dolenko's battery of joint mobility tests...four tests for the cervical spine...two for the thoracic and lumbar spine...four for the shoulder girdle...two for the elbows...three for the wrists...three for the hips...and two for the knee joints.

Illustrated descriptions and special tips:
Three plane neck movements—deceptively simple but great for bad necks...*Shoulder circles*...*Fist exercise*...*Wrist rotations*...*Elbow circles*...how to avoid contracture or age-related shortening...*The Egyptian*—an awesome shoulder loosener popular with Russian martial artists... *Russian Pool*—for super-cranking your shoulders...*Arm circles*—for all the ROM your shoulders need......*Ankle circles*...*Knee circles*..Squats...

finding the sweet spot...why deep squats are essential and how to avoid injury with correct performance...*Hula hoop*— a favorite of Russian Phys. Ed. Teachers, good for your lower back and hips...*Belly dance*—a must for martial artists...*The Cossack*—a great drill for the hip joints and your quest for splits...what *never* to do with your knees...*Split switches*—an excellent adjunct to your *Relax into Stretch* split training and simply dandy for your hips...*Spine flexion/extension*...why spine decompression is vital to spine health and mobility...*Spine rotation*...mobility drills for your spine as a top priority for rejuvenation.

How to make your body feel better than you can remember...active flexibility for sporting prowess and fewer injuries...*agonists* and *antagonists*...basic active flexibility training...how long to hold an active stretch...how to "Reach the Mark" —using the *ideomotor effect* to successfully extend your stretch...how strength coach Bill Starr develops active and passive flexibility.

How to perform the *'Pink Panther'* technique...taking advantage of the *Ukhtomsky reflex*...how one physical therapist used the Pink Panther to add a couple of feet to her hamstring stretch in one set...the partner hamstring stretch.

Is active isolated stretching any good?—the bottom line on AIS...the demographics of stretching...how and why your age and sex should dictate your choice of stretching exercises...the best techniques for young girls and boys—and what to avoid...a special warning for pregnant women...what adults should do...the elderly...and adolescents.

Stretching to help slumped shoulders...*stretch weakness* and *tight weakness*...how to address the weakness of the overstretched muscles and the tightness of their antagonists...two respected Russian regimens for better posture...understanding the vital difference between a tight and a toned muscle...the *Davis Law*...functional and dysfunctional tension.

Illustrated descriptions and special tips:
Windmill—for effectively improving the spine's rotation...*Pink Panther straight-legged situp*—the drill that can add a palm's length to your toe touch in minutes...*Bridge*—awesome for opening up the chest and improving spine extension...some warnings for those with back and wrists problems...how to dramatically improve your bridges with the *Relax into Stretch* hip flexor stretches.

'Bathtub push'—opens up the chest, great for posture and a must for a big bench press...how to develop an actively flexible spine with minimal disc loading—three tips from Russian experts...*'Ghost Pulling Knife'*—great for correcting "computer hunch"... *Shoulder dislocate with a bungee cord*—the Olympic weightlifter favorite for mutant shoulder flexibility...*Shoulder blade spread*—a popular stretch among old time strong men...*Side wall reach*...*Pink Panther knee chambers and kicks*—to dramatically improve the height and precision of your kicks...a S.W.A.T. team favorite... a unique stretching technique for high kicks from the Russian army's top hand-to-hand combat instructor...Pink Panther arabesque...add more height and power to your kicks with the *'Scissors maneuver'*.

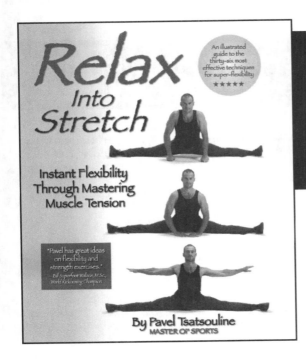

Be as Flexible as You Want to Be— Faster, Safer and Sooner

Relax into Stretch
Instant Flexibility Through Mastering Muscle Tension

By Pavel Tsatsouline

$34.95

#B14

8 1/2" x 11"   **Paperback**
150 pages   **Over 100 photos and illustrations   # B14**

An illustrated guide to the thirty-six most effective techniques for super-flexibility ★★★★★

• Own an illustrated guide to the thirty-six most effective techniques for super-flexibility
• How the secret of mastering your emotions can add immediate inches to your stretch
• How to wait out your tension—the surprising key to greater mobility and a better stretch
• How to fool your reflexes into giving you all the stretch you want
• Why *contract-relax stretching* is 267% more effective than conventional relaxed stretching
• How to breathe your way to greater flexibility
• Using the Russian technique of *Forced Relaxation* as your ultimate stretching weapon
• How to stretch when injured—faster, safer ways to heal
• Young, old, male, female—learn what stretches are best for you and what stretches to avoid
• Why excessive flexibility can be detrimental to athletic performance—and how to determine your real flexibility needs
• Plateau-busting strategies for the chronically inflexible.

"Pavel is the leading proponent of applied flexibility training at work in the field today. His ideas are dynamic and fresh. He shows the serious-minded fitness devotee another avenue of improvement. Real knowledge for real people interested in real progress."—*Marty Gallagher, WashingtonPost.com columnist, World Masters Powerlifting Champion*

"Pavel has great ideas on flexibility and strength exercises."—*Bill 'Superfoot' Wallace, M.Sc., World Kickboxing Champion*

"Conventional stretching attempts to literally elongate your tissues, which is dangerous and ineffective. Relax into Stretch simply teaches your muscles to relax into a stretch. If you compare traditional training to a messy hardware reorganization, then Relax into Stretch is an efficient software upgrade.

While stretching tissues may take years, changes in the nervous system are immediate! Your muscles will start noticeably elongating from your first **Relax into Stretch** practice—and within months you will have achieved a level of flexibility uncommon to our species."—*Pavel Tsatsouline*

Make it Easy on Yourself to be Flexible Fast!

Pavel's companion videos, *Relax into Stretch* and *Forced Relaxation*, guarantee you effortlessly master every secret for super-flexibility—so you achieve the limber, stretched-out look and high performance body you always wanted.

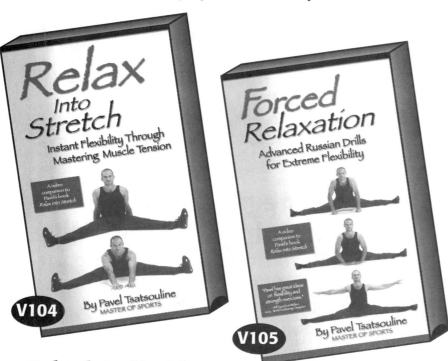

Relax into Stretch
Instant Flexibility Through Mastering Muscle Tension

By Pavel Tsatsouline

$29.95 Video

Running time: 37 minutes #V104

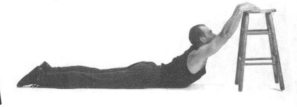

Forced Relaxation
Advanced Russian Drills for Extreme Flexibility

By Pavel Tsatsouline

$24.95 Video

Running time: 21 minutes #V105

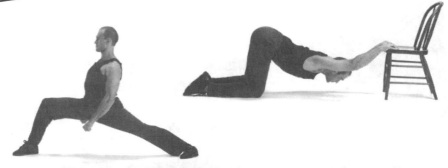

"Unleash a Shattering, Unstoppable
INTENSITY!"

What does it really take to WIN in football?

How can you turn apparent athletic mediocrity into an unstoppable force that can't stop winning?

Why do God-given talents and genetic-freaks so often fail on the field to lesser mortals?

How do you get the victory before you even step on the field?

What fail-safe training method can churn out winners, year-in, year-out, with a staggering consistency?

Enter the secret stealth weapon of modern football success, **Coach Davies**, who has helped high school, college and NFL teams turn lead into gold—and also-rans into number one—with startling frequency. In *Renegade Training for Football*, Coach Davies presents you with his full program for gridiron mastery.

"It's not a game, it's a war!" Coach Davies drills into his athletes. Extreme functional toughness, a bloody-minded brutality of purpose and a nasty-streak one mile wide defines the training mind-set.

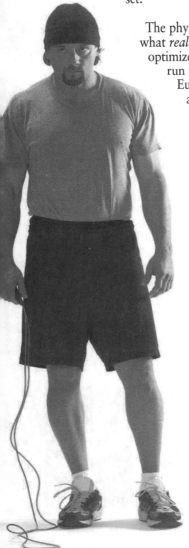

The physical program itself cuts to the core of what *really, really, really* works-in-the-trenches to optimize on-the-field performance. Techniques run the gamut from cutting-edge Eastern European to tried-and-true traditional. It's all here, from rope-skipping, stretching, hurdling, sprint set-up and Olympic lifts to esoteric Russian Kettlebells, abs-work, ladder work, jumping, tumbling and cones. A goldmine of explicit charts and racks of photographs ensure your complete grasp of how to blow past your current athletic level and ratchet up to greatness.

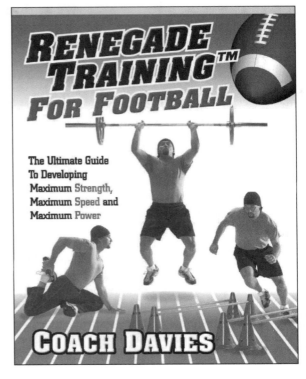

Discover everything YOU need to know for:

- **Range of Motion Development**
- **Agility Training**
- **Linear Speed Development**
- **Strength Development**
- **Work Capacity Development**
- **Spiritual Development**

We'll see YOU in the HALL OF FAME!

Renegade Training for Football
The Ultimate Guide to Developing Maximum Strength, Maximum Speed and Maximum Power

Book By Coach Davies

Paperback 225 pages 8.5" x 11"

#B21 $34.95

About the Author

Coach Davies develops comprehensive training packages for all facets and levels of football, from high school to college to the NFL. Internationally, Coach Davies has been acclaimed for his work with European and South American soccer teams.

His Renegade Training philosophy is controversial but has proved highly successful in application. Coach Davies instills a "warrior mindset" in his athletes. The result: a stand-out toughness capable of excelling in the controlled chaos and extreme stress of modern football. Physically, his athletes have consistently broken through past performance barriers to dramatically enhance their speed, strength and power.

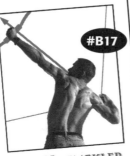

The Warrior Diet
How to Take Advantage of Undereating and Overeating

Nature's Ultimate Secret for Burning Fat, Igniting Energy and Boosting Brain Power
By Ori Hofmekler
With Diana Holtzberg

Hardcover 5 3/8" x 8 3/8", 420 pages,
Over 150 photographs and illustrations
Item #B17 **$26.95**

Eat like an emperor—and have a gladiator's body

Are you still confused about what, how and when to eat? Despite the diet books you have read and the programs you have tried, do you still find yourself lacking in energy, carrying excess body fat, and feeling physically run-down? Sexually, do you feel a shadow of your former self?

The problem, according to **Ori Hofmekler,** is that we have lost touch with the natural wisdom of our instinctual drives. We have become the slaves of our own creature comforts—scavenger/victims rather than predator/victors. When to comes to informed-choice, we lack any real sense of personal freedom. The result: ill-advised eating and lifestyle habits that leave us vulnerable to all manner of disease—not to mention obesity and sub-par performance.

The Warrior Diet presents a brilliant and far-reaching solution to our nutritional woes, based on a return to the primal power of our natural instincts.

The first step is to break the chains of our current eating habits. Drawing on a combination of ancient history and modern science, *The Warrior Diet* proves that humans are at their energetic, physical, mental and passionate best when they "undereat" during the day and "overeat" at night. Once you master this essential eating cycle, a new life of explosive vigor and vitality will be yours for the taking.

Unlike so many dietary gurus, Ori Hofmekler has personally followed his diet for over twenty-five years and is a perfect model of *the Warrior Diet's* success—the man is a human dynamo.

Not just a diet, but a whole way of life, *the Warrior Diet* encourages us to seize back the pleasures of being alive—from the most refined to the wild and raw. *The Warrior Diet* is practical, tested, and based in commonsense. Expect results!

The Warrior Diet covers all the bases. As an added bonus, discover delicious Warrior Recipes, a special Warrior Workout, and a line of Warrior Supplements—designed to give you every advantage in the transformation of your life from average to exceptional.

About Ori Hofmekler

Ori Hofmekler is a modern Renaissance man whose life has been driven by two passions: art and sports. Hofmekler's formative experience as a young man with the Israeli Special Forces, prompted a lifetime's interest in diets and fitness regimes that would optimize his physical and mental performance.

After the army, Ori attended the Bezalel Academy of Art and the Hebrew University, where he studied art and philosophy and received a degree in Human Sciences.

A world-renowned painter, best known for his controversial political satire, Ori's work has been featured in magazines worldwide, including *Time, Newsweek, Rolling Stone, People, The New Republic* as well as *Penthouse* where he was a monthly columnist for 17 years and Health Editor from 1998–2000. Ori has published two books of political art, *Hofmekler's People,* and *Hofmekler's Gallery.*

As founder, Editor-In-Chief, and Publisher of *Mind & Muscle Power,* a national men's health and fitness magazine, Ori introduced his Warrior Diet to the public in a monthly column—to immediate acclaim from readers and professionals in the health industry alike.

"In my quest for a lean, muscular body, I have seen practically every diet and suffered through most of them. It is also my business to help others with their fat loss programs. I am supremely skeptical of any eating plan or "diet" book that can't tell me how and why it works in simple language. Ori Hofmekler's *The Warrior Diet* does just this, with a logical, readable approach that provides grounding for his claims and never asks the reader to take a leap of faith. *The Warrior Diet* can be a very valuable weapon in the personal arsenal of any woman."

—**DC Maxwell, 2-time Women's Brazilian Jiu-Jitsu World Champion, Co-Owner, Maxercise Sports/Fitness Training Center and Relson Gracie Jiu-Jitsu Academy East**

"The credo that has served me well in my life and that which I tell my patients is that I only take advice from those who practice what they preach. To me, there is nothing more pathetic and laughable than to see the terrible physical condition of many of the self-proclaimed diet and fitness experts of today. Those hypocrites who do not live by their own words are not worth your time, or mine.

At the other extreme, Ori Hofmekler is the living, breathing example of a warrior. There is real strength in the sinews of his muscle. There is wisdom and power in his words. His passion for living honestly is intense and reflective of the toil of a tough army life. Yet in a fascinating and true Spartan way, his physical nature is tempered by an equal reveling in the love of art, knowledge of the classic poets, and in the drinking of fine wine with good conversation.

Welcome *The Warrior Diet* into your life and you usher in the honest and real values of a man who has truly walked the walk. He has treaded the dirt of the path that lay before you, and is thus a formidable guide to a new beginning. He is your shepherd of integrity that will lead you out of the bondage of misinformation. His approach is what I call "revolutionarily de-evolutionary". In other words, your freedom from excess body fat, flat energy levels, and poor physical performance begins with unlearning the modern ways, which have failed you, and forging a new understanding steeped in the secret traditions of the ancient Roman warrior."

—**Carlon M. Colker, M.D., F.A.C.N., author of** *The Greenwich Diet*, **CEO and Medical Director, Peak Wellness, Inc.**

"*The Warrior Diet* certainly defies so-called modern nutritional and training dogmas. Having met Ori on several occasions, I can certainly attest that he is the living proof that his system works. He maintains a ripped muscular body year round despite juggling extreme workloads and family life. His take on supplementation is refreshing as he promotes an integrated and timed approach. *The Warrior Diet* is a must read for the nutrition and training enthusiast who wishes to expand his horizons."

—**Charles Poliquin, author of** *The Poliquin Principles* **and** *Modern Trends in Strength Training*, **Three-Time Olympic Strength Coach**

"Despite its name, *The Warrior Diet* isn't about leading a Spartan lifestyle, although it is about improving quality of life. With a uniquely compelling approach, the book guides you towards the body you want by re-awakening primal instinct and biofeedback—the things that have allowed us to evolve this far.

Ironically, in a comfortable world of overindulgence, your survival may still be determined by natural selection. If this is the case, *The Warrior Diet* will be the only tool you'll need."

—**Brian Batcheldor, Science writer/researcher, National Coach, British Powerlifting Team**

"In a era of decadence, where wants and desires are virtually limitless, Ori's vision recalls an age of warriors, where success meant survival and survival was the only option. A diet of the utmost challenge from which users will reap tremendous benefits."

—**John Davies, Olympic and professional sports strength/speed coach**

"Ori Hofmekler has his finger on a deep, ancient and very visceral pulse—one that too many of us have all but forgotten. Part warrior-athlete, part philosopher-romantic, Ori not only reminds us what this innate, instinctive rhythm is all about, he also shows us how to detect and rekindle it in our own bodies. His program challenges and guides each of us to fully reclaim for ourselves the strength, sinew, energy and spirit that humans have always been meant to possess."

—**Pilar Gerasimo, Editor in Chief,** *Experience Life Magazine*

"Ori and I became friends and colleagues in 1997 when he so graciously took me under his wing as a writer for *Penthouse* Magazine and *Mind and Muscle Power*.

When I received *The Warrior Diet* in the mail I nearly burst with pride. Not only because my dear friend had finally reached his particular goal of helping others be the best they can be physically, but because I had a small role in the creation of the book. Ori enlisted my help in researching topics such as the benefits of fasting, the perfect protein, and glycogen loading. I believe in Ori's concepts because I trust him wholeheartedly and because I helped uncover the scientific data that proves them. I also live by *The Warrior Diet*, although not to the extreme that Ori does. My body continues to get tighter and more toned in all of the right places...and people marvel at my eating practices.

Read *The Warrior Diet* with an open mind. Digest the information at your own pace. Assimilate the knowledge to make it fit into your current lifestyle. You will be amazed at how much more productive and energetic you will be. Be a warrior in your own right. Your body will thank you for it."

—**Laura Moore, Science writer,** *Penthouse* **Magazine,** *IronMan* **Magazine, Body of the Month for IronMan, Sept 2001, Radio Talk Show Host** *The Health Nuts*, **author of** *Sex Heals*

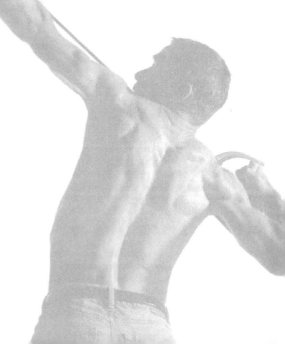

ORDERING INFORMATION

Customer Service Questions? Please call us between 9:00am–11:00pm EST Monday to Friday at 1-800-899-5111. Local and foreign customers call 513-346-4160 for orders and customer service

100% One-Year Risk-Free Guarantee. If you are not completely satisfied with any product–for any reason, no matter how long after you received it–we'll be happy to give you a prompt exchange, credit, or refund, as you wish. Simply return your purchase to us, and please let us know why you were dissatisfied–it will help us to provide better products and services in the future. *Shipping and handling fees are non-refundable.*

Telephone Orders For faster service you may place your orders by calling Toll Free 24 hours a day, 7 days a week, 365 days per year. When you call, please have your credit card ready.

1·800·899·5111
24 HOURS A DAY
FAX YOUR ORDER (866) 280-7619

Complete and mail with full payment to: Dragon Door Publications, P.O. Box 1097, West Chester, OH 45071

Please print clearly

Sold To: **A**

Name_____

Street _____

City _____

State _____ Zip _____

Day phone*_____
* Important for clarifying questions on orders

Please print clearly

SHIP TO: *(Street address for delivery)*   **B**

Name_____

Street _____

City _____

State _____ Zip _____

Email _____

ITEM #	QTY.	ITEM DESCRIPTION	ITEM PRICE	A OR B	TOTAL

HANDLING AND SHIPPING CHARGES • NO COD'S
Total Amount of Order Add:

$00.00 to $24.99 add $5.00	**$100.00 to $129.99 add $12.00**
$25.00 to $39.99 add $6.00	**$130.00 to $169.99 add $14.00**
$40.00 to $59.99 add $7.00	**$170.00 to $199.99 add $16.00**
$60.00 to $99.99 add $10.00	**$200.00 to $299.99 add $18.00**
	$300.00 and up add $20.00

Canada & Mexico add $8.00. All other countries triple U.S. charges.

Total of Goods	
Shipping Charges	
Rush Charges	
Kettlebell Shipping Charges	
OH residents add 6% sales tax	
MN residents add 6.5% sales tax	
TOTAL ENCLOSED	

METHOD OF PAYMENT ☐ CHECK ☐ M.O. ☐ MASTERCARD ☐ VISA ☐ DISCOVER ☐ AMEX

Account No. *(Please indicate all the numbers on your credit card)*   EXPIRATION DATE

☐☐☐☐ ☐☐☐☐ ☐☐☐☐ ☐☐☐☐   ☐☐/☐☐

Day Phone (   )   _____

SIGNATURE _____   DATE _____

NOTE: We ship best method available for your delivery address. Foreign orders are sent by air. Credit card or International M.O. only. For rush processing of your order, add an additional $10.00 per address. Available on money order & charge card orders only.

Errors and omissions excepted. Prices subject to change without notice.

DDP 09/02

ORDERING INFORMATION

Customer Service Questions? Please call us between 9:00am–11:00pm EST Monday to Friday at 1-800-899-5111. Local and foreign customers call 513-346-4160 for orders and customer service

100% One-Year Risk-Free Guarantee. If you are not completely satisfied with any product–for any reason, no matter how long after you received it–we'll be happy to give you a prompt exchange, credit, or refund, as you wish. Simply return your purchase to us, and please let us know why you were dissatisfied–it will help us to provide better products and services in the future. *Shipping and handling fees are non-refundable.*

Telephone Orders For faster service you may place your orders by calling Toll Free 24 hours a day, 7 days a week, 365 days per year. When you call, please have your credit card ready.

1·800·899·5111
24 HOURS A DAY
FAX YOUR ORDER (866) 280-7619

Complete and mail with full payment to: Dragon Door Publications, P.O. Box 1097, West Chester, OH 45071

Please print clearly

Sold To: **A**

Name_____

Street_____

City_____

State_____ Zip_____

Day phone*_____
* Important for clarifying questions on orders

Please print clearly

SHIP TO: *(Street address for delivery)*   **B**

Name_____

Street_____

City_____

State_____ Zip_____

Email_____

ITEM #	QTY.	ITEM DESCRIPTION	ITEM PRICE	A OR B	TOTAL

HANDLING AND SHIPPING CHARGES • NO COD'S

Total Amount of Order Add:

$00.00 to $24.99	add	$5.00	$100.00 to $129.99	add	$12.00
$25.00 to $39.99	add	$6.00	$130.00 to $169.99	add	$14.00
$40.00 to $59.99	add	$7.00	$170.00 to $199.99	add	$16.00
$60.00 to $99.99	add	$10.00	$200.00 to $299.99	add	$18.00
			$300.00 and up	add	$20.00

Canada & Mexico add $8.00. All other countries triple U.S. charges.

Total of Goods	
Shipping Charges	
Rush Charges	
Kettlebell Shipping Charges	
OH residents add 6% sales tax	
MN residents add 6.5% sales tax	
TOTAL ENCLOSED	

METHOD OF PAYMENT ☐ CHECK ☐ M.O. ☐ MASTERCARD ☐ VISA ☐ DISCOVER ☐ AMEX

Account No. *(Please indicate all the numbers on your credit card)*   EXPIRATION DATE

☐☐☐☐ ☐☐☐☐ ☐☐☐☐ ☐☐☐☐   ☐☐/☐☐

Day Phone (   ) _____

SIGNATURE _____   DATE _____

NOTE: We ship best method available for your delivery address. Foreign orders are sent by air. Credit card or International M.O. only. For rush processing of your order, add an additional $10.00 per address. Available on money order & charge card orders only.

Errors and omissions excepted. Prices subject to change without notice.